Disclaimer

The content provided in this book is for informational purposes only and is not intended to be a substitute for professional medical advice, diagnosis, or treatment. Every individual's situation is unique, and the general guidelines and recommendations may not apply to everyone. Consulting with a healthcare provider familiar with your specific situation is essential.

The information in this book is based on research and sources believed to be accurate and reliable at the time of publication. However, medical knowledge and guidelines change, and new research may emerge. Readers are encouraged to seek current information from reputable sources and consult with healthcare providers.

Any dietary or lifestyle changes, exercises, or other practices recommended in this book may carry potential risks and side effects. It is vital to consult with a healthcare provider who can assess individual risks and recommend appropriate actions.

The book is provided "as is" without any express or implied warranties. While efforts have been made to ensure accuracy and reliability, there is no guarantee that the information is error-free, complete, or suitable for any specific purpose.

Neither the authors nor publishers shall be liable for any loss, damage, injury, or adverse effects resulting from the application of the information contained in the book. Readers assume full responsibility for their use of the information.

The book may contain references to third-party websites, products, or services. These references are provided for convenience and do not constitute an endorsement or recommendation. The authors and publishers have no control over third-party content and are not responsible for its accuracy or reliability.

All content within the book is protected by copyright laws, and reproduction, distribution, or use without proper authorization is prohibited. Medical practices, dietary guidelines, and healthcare systems may vary across different cultures and regions, and readers should be aware of these variations when applying the information.

Some content in this book may be emotionally challenging or triggering for some readers. Engaging with the material with awareness of personal emotional responses and seeking support if needed is advisable.

The book is written in English and may not be accessible to all readers. Interpretations and translations should be handled with care, as nuances and specific meanings may be lost or altered.

This disclaimer emphasizes the importance of individual judgment, professional guidance, and personal responsibility when engaging with the content of the book. The information presented is intended to be informative and inspiring but must be used with caution and awareness of its limitations. By proceeding to read the book, readers acknowledge and accept the terms and conditions outlined in this disclaimer. It is the reader's responsibility to use the information within the book wisely and consult with appropriate medical and professional experts as needed.

Thank you for your understanding and happy reading!

The Chronic Kidney Disease Solution to Reclaiming Your Health

A Comprehensive Guide to Protecting and Enhancing Kidney Function Naturally and Medically

Emily J. Reynolds

Alpha Zuriel Publishing

Copyright © 2024 by **Emily J. Reynolds**

All rights reserved. No part of this publication may be reproduced, distributed, or transmitted in any form or by any means, including photocopying, recording, or other electronic or mechanical methods, without the prior written permission of the publisher, except in the case of brief quotations embodied in critical reviews and certain other noncommercial uses permitted by copyright law.

Publisher's Note: This book is designed to provide information on the subjects covered. It is sold with the understanding that the publisher is not engaged in rendering medical, health, psychological, or any other kind of personal professional services. If the reader requires personal medical, health, or other assistance or advice, a competent professional should be consulted.

The strategies, suggestions, and techniques expressed in this book are meant to be used as guidelines. They should not be used in place of professional medical advice. They are not intended to diagnose, treat, cure, or prevent any health problem - nor are they intended to replace the advice of a physician or qualified healthcare professional.

No warranties of any kind are made express or implied with respect to the contents of this book, or that any person following the advice or strategies contained herein will have a particular result. The author and publisher expressly disclaim all responsibility for any liability, loss or risk, personal or otherwise, which may be incurred as a consequence, directly or indirectly, of the use and application of any of the contents of this book.

Alpha Zuriel Publishing
Printed in the United States of America

Book Cover © 2024 Anchorage

The Chronic Kidney Disease Solution to Reclaiming Your Health -- 1st ed.

"Chronic kidney disease doesn't have to define your life. With knowledge, action, and support, you can protect your kidneys and reclaim your health."
— EMILY J. REYNOLDS

CONTENTS

WHAT IS CHRONIC KIDNEY DISEASE (CKD)? 1
   Understanding How the Kidneys Work and Why They Are So Important 3
   The Different Stages of Kidney Disease: From Mild to Severe 5
   Why Early Detection is Key to Protecting Kidney Function 7
RECOGNIZING THE SIGNS OF CHRONIC KIDNEY DISEASE ... 9
   Early Symptoms of CKD 9
   Why CKD is Often Called a "Silent" Disease 11
   Understanding How CKD Progresses 14
   Why Kidney Function Declines Over Time 16
   How to Prevent Worsening Symptoms 18
GETTING DIAGNOSED 21
   How CKD is Diagnosed 21
   Talking to Your Doctor About CKD 31
   How to Advocate for Your Kidney Health 36
MEDICATIONS TO PROTECT YOUR KIDNEY 41
   Medications commonly used for CKD 41
   Medications to Control Blood Pressure and Blood Sugar 45
   Phosphate Binders and Other Supplements to Support Kidney Health 49
   Managing Side Effects and Adjusting Medications 53
   Working with Your Doctor to Make Changes as Needed 58
LIFESTYLE CHANGES TO SUPPORT KIDNEY HEALTH 63
   The Role of Diet in Managing CKD 63
   Foods to Avoid and Foods to Include to Protect Your Kidneys 69
   The Importance of Staying Hydrated 74

    Exercise and Physical Activity 78
    Finding the Right Balance Between Activity and Rest 83
    Tips for Staying Active Without Overdoing It 87
    Reducing Stress 92
    Simple Relaxation Techniques: Meditation, Deep Breathing, and Mindfulness 96

NATURAL REMEDIES AND ALTERNATIVE THERAPIES 101

MANAGING COMMON COMPLICATIONS OF CKD 129

    High Blood Pressure 129
    Anemia and Fatigue 142
    Bone and Mineral Health 155
    Managing Fluid Retention 174

SURGICAL AND MEDICAL PROCEDURES 181

    Kidney Transplant: A Long-Term Solution 193

LONG-TERM MANAGEMENT OF CKD 217

    Regular Check-Ups and Monitoring 217
    Keeping a Healthy Routine 230
    Staying Informed About New Treatments 238

LONG-TERM MANAGEMENT OF CKD 246

    Coping with the Emotional Impact of CKD 246

PREVENTING FURTHER KIDNEY DAMAGE 269

    Preventing the Worsening of CKD 269

STORIES OF SUCCESS: PEOPLE WHO HAVE MANAGED CKD FOR YEARS 296

CONCLUSION 302

    Reclaiming Your Health with CKD 302
    Appendices 305

INTRODUCTION

WHAT IS CHRONIC KIDNEY DISEASE (CKD)?

Chronic Kidney Disease (CKD) is a long-term condition where the kidneys gradually lose their ability to function properly. This deterioration can happen over months or years, often without any noticeable symptoms in the early stages. The kidneys, two bean-shaped organs located in the lower back, play a crucial role in filtering waste products from the blood, regulating fluid and electrolyte balance, and producing hormones that h elp control blood pressure, produce red blood cells, and maintain bone health. CKD impairs these essential functions, leading to a buildup of toxins in the body, fluid retention, and other health complications.

CKD affects millions of people worldwide, making it a significant public health issue. Its progression can lead to kidney failure, also known as end-stage renal disease (ESRD), where the kidneys can no longer function without dialysis or a kidney transplant. Understanding CKD and its impact is essential for patients and healthcare providers to manage the disease effectively and slow its progression.

Understanding How the Kidneys Work and Why They Are So Important

To fully appreciate the seriousness of CKD, it's important to understand the essential functions of the kidneys. Each kidney contains approximately one million nephrons, which are the microscopic filtering units responsible for removing waste and excess substances from the blood. These nephrons work to maintain a balance of water, salts, and minerals—such as sodium, potassium, and calcium—in the bloodstream, ensuring the body's systems remain in harmony.

The kidneys also play several other vital roles:

1. Regulating Blood Pressure: They help manage blood pressure by controlling fluid levels and producing the enzyme renin, which influences blood vessel constriction.

2. Producing Hormones: The kidneys are responsible for making erythropoietin, a hormone that stimulates bone marrow to produce red blood cells.

3. Balancing Electrolytes: They keep levels of electrolytes like sodium and potassium in check, which are crucial for nerve function, muscle contraction, and maintaining the body's fluid balance.

4. Excreting Waste: As blood flows through the kidneys, toxins and waste products from metabolism, such as urea and

creatinine, are filtered out and excreted in urine. This process prevents toxic buildup that could harm organs and tissues.

5.   Bone Health: Kidneys convert Vitamin D into its active form, helping to regulate calcium and phosphorus levels, which are vital for strong bones.

The Different Stages of Kidney Disease: From Mild to Severe

CKD is classified into five stages based on the level of kidney function, specifically measured by the glomerular filtration rate (GFR), which estimates how much blood is filtered by the kidneys each minute. The lower the GFR, the more severe the kidney damage. The five stages of CKD are:

• **Stage 1 (Mild Kidney Damage, Normal GFR)**: In this stage, kidney function is still normal, but there may be structural damage, such as protein in the urine (proteinuria) or other signs of kidney damage. GFR is at 90 mL/min or higher.

• **Stage 2 (Mild Kidney Damage, GFR Decline)**: A slight decrease in GFR (60-89 mL/min) is present, indicating mild loss of kidney function. At this point, most people have no symptoms but may show signs of damage, such as elevated blood pressure or proteinuria.

• **Stage 3 (Moderate CKD)**: Divided into 3a (GFR 45-59 mL/min) and 3b (GFR 30-44 mL/min), this stage indicates moderate loss of kidney function. Symptoms may begin to appear, including fatigue, fluid retention, and abnormal lab values for electrolytes or waste products.

• **Stage 4 (Severe CKD)**: GFR drops to 15-29 mL/min, indicating severe damage to the kidneys. Symptoms become more pronounced, with swelling, high blood pressure, and signs of waste accumulation in the body (uremia).

- **Stage 5 (End-Stage Renal Disease):** At this stage, GFR falls below 15 mL/min, meaning the kidneys have nearly or completely stopped functioning. Without dialysis or a transplant, toxic substances will build up in the body, leading to life-threatening complications.

Why Early Detection is Key to Protecting Kidney Function

Early detection of CKD can be lifesaving. Many people with CKD don't experience noticeable symptoms until the disease has progressed to an advanced stage, making routine screening essential, especially for those at higher risk—such as individuals with diabetes, hypertension, or a family history of kidney disease.

Regular testing of kidney function, including blood tests for GFR and urine tests for protein, can identify CKD before it causes significant harm. Early diagnosis allows for timely intervention to slow or stop the progression of the disease through lifestyle changes, medication, and careful monitoring. Patients diagnosed early can take steps to control blood pressure, manage blood sugar levels, and adopt a kidney-friendly diet to protect remaining kidney function.

CHAPTER ONE

RECOGNIZING THE SIGNS OF CHRONIC KIDNEY DISEASE

Early Symptoms of CKD

Fatigue, Swelling, and High Blood Pressure: What to Look For

In the early stages of Chronic Kidney Disease (CKD), the symptoms can be subtle or mistaken for other health issues. However, as the disease progresses, certain signs become more noticeable. Three of the most common symptoms that indicate kidney problems are fatigue, swelling, and high blood pressure. Recognizing these can be key to catching CKD early.

Fatigue
One of the earliest and most common symptoms of CKD is feeling unusually tired or exhausted, even with adequate rest. This happens because damaged kidneys are less able to filter toxins and waste from the blood, leading to a buildup that can make you feel sluggish and weak. Additionally, CKD often

leads to anemia, a condition where the body doesn't produce enough red blood cells, which can worsen fatigue.

Swelling (Edema)

As kidney function declines, the body starts to retain fluids that the kidneys can no longer properly filter out. This leads to swelling, known as edema, which is commonly seen in the legs, ankles, feet, and sometimes the hands or face. Swelling can cause discomfort, make shoes feel tight, or lead to weight gain due to fluid retention. The buildup of fluid can also affect the lungs, leading to shortness of breath.

High Blood Pressure

The kidneys play a key role in regulating blood pressure. When they aren't working well, they can cause blood pressure to rise. High blood pressure (hypertension) is both a symptom and a cause of CKD, creating a vicious cycle: kidney damage leads to high blood pressure, which in turn can worsen kidney function. High blood pressure is often silent, with no noticeable symptoms, but if left untreated, it can lead to serious complications such as heart disease or stroke.

Together, these symptoms—fatigue, swelling, and high blood pressure—are important warning signs. If they appear, it's crucial to consult a healthcare provider to evaluate kidney function and begin appropriate treatment.

Why CKD is Often Called a "Silent" Disease

Chronic Kidney Disease is often referred to as a "silent" disease because in the early stages, there are usually no obvious symptoms. The kidneys are highly efficient organs, and they can continue to function with as little as 10% of their capacity before noticeable problems arise. This means that people can lose significant kidney function without realizing it.

By the time symptoms like fatigue, swelling, or changes in urination patterns appear, the disease may have already progressed to a more advanced stage. Many individuals remain unaware of their condition until routine blood or urine tests show abnormal kidney function, or until complications like high blood pressure or anemia develop.

The silent nature of CKD makes it crucial for those at higher risk—such as individuals with diabetes, high blood pressure, or a family history of kidney disease—to undergo regular screenings. Catching the disease early through these tests can allow for interventions that slow its progression and help preserve kidney function.

How to Catch Kidney Problems Before They Become Serious

Because Chronic Kidney Disease (CKD) often shows no symptoms in its early stages, detecting it before it becomes serious requires proactive measures. The key to catching kidney problems early lies in regular screenings, especially for those at higher risk. Here's how you can spot potential issues before they lead to severe damage:

1. Routine Blood Tests

A blood test measuring the levels of creatinine, a waste product filtered by the kidneys, can provide an important clue. From this, doctors can estimate your Glomerular Filtration Rate (GFR), which indicates how well your kidneys are functioning. A lower GFR suggests reduced kidney function. Regular monitoring of GFR is crucial in identifying kidney problems before they worsen.

2. Urine Tests

Protein in the urine (proteinuria) is one of the earliest signs of kidney damage. A simple urine test can detect the presence of proteins like albumin, which should normally be retained by the kidneys. If proteins are found in the urine, it could indicate that the kidneys' filtering system is compromised.

3. Blood Pressure Monitoring

High blood pressure is both a cause and a result of CKD. Regular monitoring of your blood pressure is important because elevated blood pressure can damage the kidneys over time. If you consistently have high readings, it may be a sign that your kidneys are under strain, even if you don't feel unwell.

4. Pay Attention to Changes in Urination

While CKD is often silent, subtle changes in your urination patterns may provide early warning signs. Look out for frequent urination, especially at night, or changes in the color or appearance of urine, such as it becoming foamy (indicating proteinuria). Any unusual changes should be reported to your healthcare provider.

5. Regular Checkups if You're High-Risk

Those with conditions like diabetes, hypertension, or a family history of kidney disease should get regular kidney function tests. This includes yearly screenings for kidney health, even if you don't have any symptoms. Early intervention can slow or prevent the progression of CKD.

Catching CKD early gives patients the best chance at slowing its progress, managing symptoms, and maintaining a better quality of life.

Understanding How CKD Progresses

Chronic Kidney Disease (CKD) does not happen all at once—it progresses in stages, with kidney function gradually worsening over time. Understanding how CKD progresses is essential for both patients and healthcare providers, as it helps guide treatment decisions and lifestyle changes that can slow the decline of kidney function.

The Stages of CKD: What They Mean for Your Health

CKD is classified into five stages based on how well the kidneys filter waste from the blood. This filtering ability is measured by the Glomerular Filtration Rate (GFR), which estimates the amount of blood that passes through the kidneys per minute. As CKD advances, GFR decreases, and kidney function worsens.

- **Stage 1:** In this early stage, the kidneys still function normally or close to normally, but signs of kidney damage, such as protein in the urine or physical changes in the kidneys, may be present. The GFR is 90 mL/min or higher. At this point, lifestyle changes and close monitoring are important to prevent further damage.

- **Stage 2:** At this stage, there is a mild reduction in kidney function, with a GFR between 60 and 89 mL/min. Patients may not experience any noticeable symptoms, but kidney damage is detectable. Careful management of underlying conditions, like diabetes or high blood pressure, is essential.

- **Stage 3:** Divided into two parts, Stage 3a (GFR 45-59 mL/min) and Stage 3b (GFR 30-44 mL/min), this stage represents moderate CKD. Symptoms such as fatigue, swelling, and changes in urination may begin to appear. At this stage, it's important to control blood pressure, monitor diet, and take steps to protect kidney health.

- **Stage 4:** With a GFR between 15 and 29 mL/min, Stage 4 indicates severe kidney damage. Symptoms become more pronounced, and patients may experience significant fatigue, fluid retention, and higher blood pressure. At this stage, healthcare providers typically start preparing patients for the possibility of dialysis or a kidney transplant in the near future.

- **Stage 5:** Also known as End-Stage Renal Disease (ESRD), Stage 5 occurs when GFR drops below 15 mL/min. The kidneys can no longer filter waste effectively, and dialysis or a kidney transplant becomes necessary to sustain life. Symptoms can be severe, including nausea, vomiting, shortness of breath, and confusion due to the buildup of toxins in the blood.

Understanding the stage of CKD you are in, helps to guide you through the treatment and lifestyle adjustments to manage the disease.

Why Kidney Function Declines Over Time

Kidney function declines gradually in people with Chronic Kidney Disease (CKD) due to several underlying factors. Over time, damage to the kidneys accumulates, making it harder for these organs to effectively filter waste and maintain balance in the body. Let's explore why this happens:

1. Ongoing Damage to Kidney Cells

The kidneys are made up of millions of tiny filtering units called nephrons. When you have CKD, various factors—such as high blood pressure, high blood sugar (in diabetes), or inflammation—can damage these nephrons. Once damaged, nephrons cannot regenerate. As more and more nephrons stop working, the kidneys lose their ability to function properly.

2. Scarring of Kidney Tissue

As CKD progresses, inflammation within the kidneys can lead to the formation of scar tissue (a process called fibrosis). This scarring further reduces kidney function by blocking the proper flow of blood and the filtration process. Over time, this damage spreads and worsens, causing further declines in kidney efficiency.

3. Increased Workload on Remaining Nephrons

As more nephrons become damaged or die, the remaining healthy nephrons have to work harder to compensate. This increased workload puts stress on the surviving nephrons, which accelerates their decline. Eventually, even the remaining functional nephrons can become overworked and damaged, further speeding up the loss of kidney function.

4. Underlying Health Conditions

Certain conditions, like high blood pressure and diabetes, are major contributors to CKD progression. These diseases can cause continuous strain on the kidneys, leading to further deterioration. High blood pressure, for example, causes damage to the blood vessels in the kidneys, reducing their ability to filter blood effectively. Similarly, uncontrolled blood sugar in diabetes can lead to the gradual destruction of kidney tissue.

5. Aging

As people age, kidney function naturally declines. However, in people with CKD, this process happens much faster. The kidneys may not be able to keep up with the body's needs, especially if other health problems are present. The combined effects of aging and CKD make it even more difficult for the kidneys to maintain normal function.

When you understand why kidney function declines over time, it can help you or any patient take proactive steps to manage their condition, including controlling blood pressure, managing diabetes, and following a kidney-friendly diet. These efforts can help slow the progression of the disease.

How to Prevent Worsening Symptoms

Preventing the worsening of Chronic Kidney Disease (CKD) requires active management of the condition through lifestyle changes, medications, and regular monitoring. While CKD is a progressive disease, its advancement can often be slowed down by adopting the right habits and interventions. Here are key strategies to help prevent worsening symptoms:

1. Control Blood Pressure

High blood pressure is one of the leading causes of kidney damage. Keeping blood pressure under control is essential for protecting kidney function. Patients with CKD should aim to keep their blood pressure below 130/80 mm Hg. This can be achieved by taking prescribed medications, such as ACE inhibitors or ARBs, and making lifestyle changes like reducing salt intake, exercising regularly, and maintaining a healthy weight.

2. Manage Blood Sugar Levels

For people with diabetes, high blood sugar can damage the blood vessels in the kidneys, leading to further loss of function. Monitoring and controlling blood sugar levels can significantly reduce the risk of kidney damage. This includes following a diabetes-friendly diet, taking insulin or oral medications as prescribed, and regularly checking blood sugar levels.

3. Follow a Kidney-Friendly Diet

Diet plays a crucial role in managing CKD and preventing worsening symptoms. A kidney-friendly diet typically involves limiting salt, potassium, and phosphorus intake, which helps reduce strain on the kidneys. Patients should also aim for a balanced diet rich in fruits, vegetables, whole grains, and lean proteins, while avoiding processed foods and those high in sodium. It's also important to limit protein intake to avoid overworking the kidneys.

4. Stay Hydrated, But Don't Overdo It

While staying hydrated is important for kidney health, drinking excessive amounts of water can sometimes strain the kidneys, especially in more advanced stages of CKD. It's important to follow your healthcare provider's recommendations on how much fluid you should drink each day, depending on the stage of your disease and other health factors.

5. Avoid Nonsteroidal Anti-Inflammatory Drugs (NSAIDs)

Over-the-counter pain relievers like ibuprofen and naproxen can worsen kidney damage in people with CKD. These drugs reduce blood flow to the kidneys and can accelerate the progression of the disease. It's important to avoid these medications and consult your healthcare provider for safer alternatives.

6. Stay Active and Maintain a Healthy Weight

Regular physical activity helps maintain overall health and can improve blood pressure control, reduce the risk of diabetes, and improve heart health—all of which are critical for slowing CKD progression. Aim for at least 30 minutes of moderate exercise, like walking or cycling, most days of the week. Additionally, maintaining a healthy weight can reduce stress on the kidneys and improve kidney function.

7. Quit Smoking

Smoking damages blood vessels, reduces blood flow to the kidneys, and worsens kidney function. Quitting smoking can slow down the progression of CKD and reduce the risk of cardiovascular diseases, which are common in people with kidney disease.

8. Regular Monitoring and Follow-up

Regular checkups with your healthcare provider are crucial for monitoring the progression of CKD and adjusting treatment plans as needed. This includes blood and urine tests to monitor kidney function, blood pressure checks, and discussions about medications and lifestyle changes. Staying on top of these appointments can catch any worsening symptoms early and allow for timely intervention.

By taking these steps, patients can help prevent the
worsening of CKD symptoms and maintain a higher quality of life for a longer period. Slowing the progression of CKD may also delay or avoid the need for dialysis or a kidney transplant.

CHAPTER TWO

GETTING DIAGNOSED

How CKD is Diagnosed

Key Tests: Blood Tests (Creatinine and GFR), Urine Tests, and Imaging

Diagnosing and monitoring Chronic Kidney Disease (CKD) requires a combination of blood, urine, and imaging tests. Each of these tests provides valuable insights into how well the kidneys are functioning and whether any damage has occurred. Here's an overview of the key tests used in diagnosing CKD:

1. Blood Tests (Creatinine and GFR)
Creatinine Test:
Creatinine is a waste product that muscles produce as part of normal metabolism. Healthy kidneys filter creatinine out of the blood and remove it through urine. However, when the kidneys aren't functioning properly, creatinine levels in the

blood start to rise, indicating that the kidneys aren't effectively filtering waste.

To measure how well the kidneys are working, doctors perform a blood test to check your serum creatinine level. Higher-than-normal creatinine levels suggest impaired kidney function.

Glomerular Filtration Rate (GFR):

The creatinine test results are used to calculate your Glomerular Filtration Rate (GFR), which is a key indicator of kidney health. GFR measures how much blood the kidneys filter each minute and is adjusted for factors like age, sex, and race.

A normal GFR is around 90 mL/min or higher, depending on your age, but as kidney function declines, GFR drops. Based on your GFR, CKD is classified into five stages, with Stage 1 indicating mild kidney damage and Stage 5 representing kidney failure. A GFR below 60 mL/min for three months or more usually confirms the presence of CKD.

2. Urine Tests
Urinalysis:

A urine test is another essential tool in diagnosing CKD. One of the earliest signs of kidney damage is protein leaking into the urine. Healthy kidneys typically don't allow much protein to pass into the urine, but when the kidneys are damaged, they can lose their ability to keep protein in the blood.

A simple dipstick urine test can detect protein (albumin) in the urine. If protein is found, further tests will measure how much is present.

Urine Albumin-to-Creatinine Ratio (UACR):

One common urine test to measure kidney damage is the Urine Albumin-to-Creatinine Ratio (UACR). This test compares the amount of albumin (a type of protein) in the urine to the level of creatinine. A UACR of 30 mg/g or higher may indicate early kidney damage and is used to monitor how well treatment is working. Regular urine tests are critical for tracking CKD progression, especially for individuals with diabetes or high blood pressure, where protein leakage is common.

3. Imaging Tests
Ultrasound:

An ultrasound is a non-invasive imaging test that uses sound waves to create pictures of the kidneys. It can detect structural abnormalities like kidney stones, cysts, or tumors, which could be affecting kidney function. Ultrasounds can also reveal blockages in the urinary tract or changes in kidney size, which are often signs of CKD.

CT Scan or MRI:

For a more detailed view, doctors may recommend a CT scan or MRI. These tests provide clearer images of the kidneys and surrounding structures. A CT scan or MRI can help detect scarring, blockages, or masses that an ultrasound might miss. These imaging tests are particularly useful in diagnosing causes of CKD that may not be apparent through blood or urine tests alone.

Kidney Biopsy (in some cases):

In certain cases, doctors may suggest a kidney biopsy. This involves taking a small sample of kidney tissue to examine under a microscope. A biopsy can provide detailed information about the type of kidney disease, the extent of damage, and the likely cause, helping doctors tailor the treatment plan more effectively.

After combining the results of these blood, urine, and imaging tests, healthcare providers can diagnose CKD, determine its severity, and decide on the best course of treatment to slow the disease's progression and manage symptoms.

What the Numbers Mean: Understanding Your Kidney Function Results

When you're diagnosed with Chronic Kidney Disease (CKD), your healthcare provider will regularly monitor specific test results to assess how well your kidneys are functioning. Understanding what these numbers mean can help you stay informed about your condition and the steps you need to take to manage it.

1. Creatinine Levels

Creatinine is a waste product from muscle activity, and healthy kidneys remove it from the bloodstream. If your kidneys aren't working well, creatinine builds up in your blood. The normal range for serum creatinine varies depending on age, gender, and muscle mass, but in general:
- For men: 0.6 to 1.2 mg/dL
- For women: 0.5 to 1.1 mg/dL

Higher levels of creatinine in your blood suggest that your kidneys are not filtering waste as effectively as they should. This result is often used alongside your Glomerular Filtration Rate (GFR) to get a clearer picture of your kidney health.

2. Glomerular Filtration Rate (GFR)

Your GFR is one of the most important numbers you'll encounter when managing CKD. GFR measures how much blood your kidneys filter every minute. It's calculated using your creatinine level, age, gender, and race.

The GFR results are typically broken down into the following categories:

- **90 mL/min or higher:** Normal kidney function, but if there are signs of kidney damage (like protein in the urine), this may indicate Stage 1 CKD.
- **60 to 89 mL/min:** Slightly reduced kidney function. If combined with other signs of damage, this is classified as Stage 2 CKD.
- **30 to 59 mL/min:** Moderate reduction in kidney function (Stage 3 CKD). This is where symptoms like fatigue or swelling may begin to appear.
- **15 to 29 mL/min:** Severe reduction in kidney function (Stage 4 CKD). At this stage, you may need to start preparing for dialysis or a kidney transplant.
- **Below 15 mL/min:** Kidney failure (Stage 5 CKD), also known as End-Stage Renal Disease (ESRD), requiring dialysis or a transplant to survive.

Tracking your GFR over time helps your doctor determine how quickly your kidney function is declining and what treatments may be necessary to slow the progression.

3. Urine Albumin-to-Creatinine Ratio (UACR)

The UACR test compares the amount of albumin (a type of protein) to creatinine in your urine. This is a key indicator of how much protein is leaking from your kidneys, which normally do not allow protein to pass into the urine. A high UACR means that your kidneys are damaged and leaking protein.

- A normal UACR is less than 30 mg/g.
- A UACR between 30 and 300 mg/g suggests early kidney disease.
- A UACR over 300 mg/g indicates more severe kidney damage.

Regular monitoring of your UACR can show how well your kidneys are responding to treatment, especially if you have conditions like diabetes or hypertension, which often cause protein leakage.

4. Blood Pressure

High blood pressure is both a cause and a result of CKD. Monitoring your blood pressure regularly is essential because elevated levels can accelerate kidney damage. For most people with CKD, the target blood pressure is below 130/80 mm Hg. Controlling blood pressure with lifestyle changes and medication is key to slowing down CKD progression.

5. Other Blood Test Results

In addition to creatinine and GFR, your doctor may also check levels of other substances in your blood to monitor your overall health:

- Electrolytes (such as sodium, potassium, and calcium) are closely regulated by the kidneys. Imbalances can indicate worsening kidney function.
- Blood Urea Nitrogen (BUN) measures another waste product filtered by the kidneys. High levels may indicate kidney dysfunction.
- Hemoglobin and red blood cell counts are checked because CKD can cause anemia, leading to fatigue and other symptoms.

By understanding these key test results, you'll be better equipped to work with your healthcare provider in managing CKD and taking steps to protect your kidney function.

Why It's Important to Monitor Your Blood Pressure and Blood Sugar

Managing Chronic Kidney Disease (CKD) isn't just about focusing on kidney health. It also involves closely monitoring two major factors that can both cause and worsen kidney damage: blood pressure and blood sugar levels. Keeping these under control can help slow the progression of CKD and prevent further damage to your kidneys.

1. Blood Pressure and CKD

High blood pressure (hypertension) is one of the leading causes of CKD and also a common complication of the disease. Here's why it's important to keep it in check:

- **How High Blood Pressure Affects the Kidneys:** Blood pressure refers to the force of blood pushing against the walls of your blood vessels. When this pressure is too high, it can damage the tiny blood vessels (glomeruli) in the kidneys. These blood vessels are responsible for filtering waste and excess fluids from the blood. Over time, high blood pressure causes these vessels to weaken and narrow, leading to a decline in kidney function.

- **CKD and Hypertension: A Vicious Cycle:** CKD and hypertension often fuel each other. Damaged kidneys have trouble controlling blood pressure, which can then rise and cause further kidney damage. This cycle can lead to faster disease progression if not carefully managed.

- **Monitoring and Managing Blood Pressure:** For people with CKD, the target blood pressure is typically below 130/80 mm Hg. Regular monitoring, lifestyle changes, and medications such as ACE inhibitors or ARBs can help control blood pressure and reduce stress on the kidneys. Managing your salt intake, exercising regularly, and avoiding excessive alcohol are important lifestyle adjustments that can make a big difference.

2. Blood Sugar and CKD

For people with diabetes, keeping blood sugar levels under control is essential to protecting kidney health. High blood sugar can damage the kidneys over time, leading to CKD. Here's how:

- **How High Blood Sugar Affects the Kidneys:** Elevated blood sugar levels damage the blood vessels in the kidneys, leading to a condition called diabetic nephropathy. This damage occurs gradually, making it harder for the kidneys to filter waste. Excess sugar in the bloodstream can also cause scarring and narrowing of the kidney's filtering units, which leads to reduced kidney function.

- **Diabetes and CKD:** Diabetes is one of the most common causes of CKD. People with poorly controlled diabetes are at a higher risk of developing kidney disease and experiencing a faster decline in kidney function. Maintaining normal blood sugar levels is crucial in preventing kidney damage.

- **Monitoring and Managing Blood Sugar:** For those with diabetes, regular blood sugar monitoring is critical. The goal is to maintain an A1C level (a measure of average blood sugar levels over the past 2-3 months) below 7%, though individual targets may vary depending on other health factors. Managing your diet, staying physically active, and following your prescribed medication or insulin regimen are essential for keeping blood sugar in a healthy range.

3. Why It's Critical to Monitor Both

Blood pressure and blood sugar are closely linked to kidney health. Poorly controlled blood pressure and blood sugar levels can accelerate kidney damage, leading to faster progression of CKD. By monitoring these regularly, you can catch any changes early and make the necessary adjustments to your treatment plan.

Managing both factors together through a combination of medication, lifestyle changes, and regular doctor visits is key to slowing the progression of CKD and protecting your kidney function for as long as possible.

Talking to Your Doctor About CKD

Questions to Ask to Understand Your Diagnosis and Treatment Options

Being diagnosed with Chronic Kidney Disease (CKD) can be overwhelming, but asking the right questions can help you understand your condition and feel more in control of your treatment. When you meet with your healthcare provider, consider discussing the following key areas to ensure you have a clear understanding of your diagnosis and what comes next.

1. What Stage of CKD Do I Have?

Understanding the stage of CKD you're in is essential because it determines how much kidney function you have left and what steps need to be taken next. Ask your doctor:

- . What is my Glomerular Filtration Rate (GFR)?
- . What stage of CKD am I in, and what does that mean for my health?
- . How quickly is my kidney function declining, and what can I do to slow the progression?

2. What Is Causing My Kidney Disease?

CKD can have several causes, such as diabetes, high blood pressure, or genetic factors. Knowing the underlying cause is important for managing the disease and preventing further damage.

- What is the primary cause of my CKD?

- . Are there other factors that might be contributing to my kidney damage?
- How can I manage these causes or reduce their impact on my kidneys?

3. What Treatment Options Are Available?

There are many treatment options depending on your stage of CKD. These treatments can range from lifestyle changes and medications to managing symptoms or slowing the disease's progression.

- What treatments are recommended for my stage of CKD?
- Are there specific medications I should take to manage symptoms like high blood pressure or swelling?
- What lifestyle changes should I make to support my kidney health?
- Will I need dialysis in the future, and when I start preparing for that?

4. How Will You Monitor My Condition?

CKD requires ongoing monitoring to assess the effectiveness of treatment and detect any worsening of kidney function. Ask your doctor:

- How often will I need blood and urine tests to monitor my kidney function?
- What specific results or symptoms should I be watching for between checkups?
- What will you be looking for in my test results to decide if my treatment needs to change?

5. How Can I Manage Other Health Conditions Alongside CKD?

Many people with CKD also have other chronic conditions like diabetes, high blood pressure, or heart disease. Coordinating the treatment for these conditions is critical to overall health.

- How can I manage my other health conditions (like diabetes or high blood pressure) in a way that supports my kidney health?
- Are there medications I should avoid that could harm my kidneys?
- Can you recommend a diet that works for both my kidney health and other health issues?

6. What Are the Risks of My Current Medications?

Certain medications can impact kidney health, either by overloading the kidneys or by interacting with CKD treatments.

- Are any of my current medications harmful to my kidneys?
- Do I need to adjust any of my medications due to my CKD diagnosis?
- Are there medications I should be cautious about taking, such as over-the-counter pain relievers like ibuprofen?

7. What Can I Do to Improve My Kidney Health?

Beyond medications, there are many things you can do to support your kidneys and overall well-being. Ask about lifestyle changes and preventive strategies.

- What dietary changes should I make to protect my kidneys?
- How can I incorporate physical activity into my routine without overburdening my kidneys?

- Are there specific supplements or vitamins that can help?

8. What Should I Expect Going Forward?

CKD is a progressive disease, and understanding the long-term outlook is important for managing expectations and making plans.

- How will my condition likely change over time?
- What are the warning signs that my condition is worsening, and what should I do if I notice them?
- At what point might I need dialysis or a kidney transplant, and what are the signs that these treatments might be necessary?

9. How Can I Get Emotional or Psychological Support?

A CKD diagnosis can be emotionally challenging. Managing a chronic illness often brings stress, anxiety, or depression.

- Can you recommend support groups or counseling services for CKD patients?
- What resources are available for helping me cope with the emotional aspects of living with CKD?
- Are there specific strategies for managing the stress of this diagnosis?

10. How Can I Stay Informed About My Condition?

The more you know about CKD, the better equipped you'll be to manage your health. Ask for resources to help you stay informed.

- Are there educational materials or trusted websites where I can learn more about CKD?

- How can I stay updated on new treatments or advances in kidney care?
- Is there a patient portal or way for me to track my test results and progress between appointments?

By asking these questions, you can better understand your diagnosis, treatment options, and what steps to take to preserve your kidney health. Don't hesitate to seek clarity from your healthcare provider, as staying informed is one of the most important ways to manage CKD effectively.

How to Advocate for Your Kidney Health

Living with Chronic Kidney Disease (CKD) requires not only medical treatment but also self-advocacy. Being proactive about your health and taking charge of your care is essential in managing the disease and improving your quality of life. Advocacy means understanding your condition, communicating clearly with your healthcare team, and ensuring you get the right treatments and support. Here's how you can advocate for your kidney health:

1. Stay Informed About Your Condition

Knowledge is power, especially when it comes to managing CKD. The more you understand your disease, the more effectively you can communicate with your doctors and make informed decisions.

- Learn About CKD: Read reputable sources, ask your healthcare provider for educational materials, and stay up-to-date with new treatments and advances in kidney care. This knowledge can help you understand your diagnosis, test results, and treatment options.
- Ask Questions: Don't hesitate to ask your doctor to explain anything you don't understand, whether it's medical terms, treatment plans, or the potential side effects of medications. Keep a list of questions for your appointments so you can cover everything that's important to you.

2. Build a Strong Relationship with Your Healthcare Team

Your healthcare team plays a vital role in managing your CKD, and maintaining open, honest communication with them is key. This relationship helps ensure you receive personalized care that meets your needs.

- Be Open About Symptoms and Concerns: Let your healthcare provider know about any new symptoms or changes in your condition, even if they seem minor. This helps them adjust your treatment as necessary.

- Prepare for Appointments: Bring a list of your medications, supplements, and any symptoms you've experienced. Preparing in advance ensures you make the most of your time with your doctor and helps them provide better care.

- Get a Second Opinion: If you're unsure about a diagnosis or treatment plan, don't hesitate to seek a second opinion. This can give you confidence that you're on the right path or introduce new perspectives on managing your condition.

3. Keep Track of Your Health Data

Monitoring your health data can help you take control of your CKD and detect any changes early. This includes keeping track of your test results, symptoms, medications, and lifestyle changes.

- Monitor Blood Pressure and Blood Sugar: If you have high blood pressure or diabetes, regularly checking these levels at home can help you stay in control. High blood pressure and blood sugar levels can worsen CKD, so catching these changes early can make a big difference.

- **Track Your Kidney Function:** Keep a record of your blood test results, especially your GFR and creatinine levels. This helps you understand how your kidneys are doing over time and allows you to spot trends that may indicate a need for adjustments in treatment.
- **Maintain a Symptom Journal:** Write down any new symptoms, changes in urination, or other health concerns. This journal can be a useful tool during medical appointments to give your doctor a clear picture of how you're doing.

4. Advocate for Yourself in Medical Settings

When it comes to managing CKD, you are your own best advocate. Speak up for your needs and preferences, especially in medical settings where important decisions about your treatment are being made.

- **Communicate Your Preferences:** If you have specific preferences about your treatment—whether it's avoiding certain medications, trying lifestyle changes first, or exploring alternative therapies—make sure your doctor knows. Clear communication can ensure your treatment aligns with your values and goals.
- **Know Your Rights:** As a patient, you have the right to be fully informed about your diagnosis, treatment options, and any potential risks. You also have the right to be involved in all decisions about your care. Don't be afraid to ask for explanations or alternatives if something doesn't feel right.

5. Build a Support Network

Having a network of support is essential when managing a chronic illness like CKD. Whether it's family, friends, or a support group, these people can provide emotional and practical help when you need it most.

- Connect with a Support Group: Joining a CKD support group can be a great way to share experiences, learn from others, and feel less isolated. Many people find it helpful to talk to others who are going through similar challenges, and it can provide a safe space to express concerns and get advice.
- Lean on Loved Ones: Don't hesitate to ask friends or family for help, whether it's attending doctor appointments with you, assisting with day-to-day tasks, or providing emotional support. A strong support system can make a huge difference in your overall well-being.

6. Make Lifestyle Changes that Support Kidney Health

Taking control of your daily habits can significantly impact your kidney health. Even small changes in diet, exercise, and stress management can help slow the progression of CKD.

- Adopt a Kidney-Friendly Diet: Work with a dietitian or your doctor to create a diet plan that reduces stress on your kidneys. This often includes cutting down on salt, potassium, and phosphorus, while eating more fruits, vegetables, and lean proteins.
- Stay Active: Regular exercise can help control blood pressure, manage weight, and improve overall health. Aim for activities that are gentle on your body, like walking or swimming.
- Quit Smoking: Smoking can damage blood vessels and worsen CKD. Quitting smoking is one of the best things you can do to protect your kidneys and improve your overall health.

7. Stay Engaged in Your Treatment Plan

It's essential to stay actively involved in managing your CKD. Regular follow-ups, taking prescribed medications as directed, and making necessary lifestyle adjustments are all important.

- Follow Your Doctor's Recommendations: Take medications as prescribed and make any lifestyle adjustments recommended by your healthcare team. Consistency is key in slowing the progression of CKD.
- Attend Regular Checkups: Don't skip appointments or lab tests. Regular monitoring is crucial for adjusting your treatment plan and preventing complications.
- Ask for Updated Information: CKD treatment options are always evolving. Ask your doctor about new medications, procedures, or lifestyle interventions that may help manage your condition more effectively.

By being proactive and advocating for yourself, you can play a critical role in managing your CKD and protecting your kidney health. It's about becoming an active participant in your care, staying informed, and making choices that align with your health goals.

CHAPTER THREE

MEDICATIONS TO PROTECT YOUR KIDNEY

Medications commonly used for CKD

ACE Inhibitors and ARBs: How They Help Protect Kidney Function

One of the key strategies in managing Chronic Kidney Disease (CKD) is to slow down the progression of kidney damage, and medications like ACE inhibitors and ARBs play a vital role in this effort. These medications, commonly prescribed for people with high blood pressure or diabetes, have been shown to help protect kidney function by controlling blood pressure and reducing strain on the kidneys.

What Are ACE Inhibitors and ARBs?
- ACE Inhibitors (Angiotensin-Converting Enzyme Inhibitors): These medications work by blocking the enzyme that produces angiotensin II, a substance that narrows blood vessels. When blood vessels narrow, it increases blood pressure and forces the heart and kidneys to work harder. By preventing

the production of angiotensin II, ACE inhibitors help relax blood vessels, lower blood pressure, and reduce the pressure on the kidneys.

- ARBs (Angiotensin II Receptor Blockers): Like ACE inhibitors, ARBs affect angiotensin II, but they work by blocking the action of this substance rather than its production. Angiotensin II binds to specific receptors in the blood vessels, causing them to tighten. ARBs block this binding, allowing blood vessels to stay relaxed and lowering blood pressure in the process.

Both ACE inhibitors and ARBs are effective in reducing blood pressure and protecting the kidneys. They are often used as first-line treatments for people with CKD, particularly those with diabetes or hypertension, two conditions that can significantly worsen kidney damage.

How Do These Medications Protect the Kidneys?

ACE inhibitors and ARBs have a unique protective effect on the kidneys beyond simply lowering blood pressure. Here's how they help:

- Reduce Pressure in the Kidneys: In people with CKD, high blood pressure increases the force with which blood flows into the kidneys. This pressure can damage the tiny filtering units (glomeruli) within the kidneys, leading to scarring and a reduction in kidney function over time. By lowering blood pressure, ACE inhibitors and ARBs reduce the strain on the glomeruli, helping to preserve kidney function.

- Decrease Protein in the Urine (Proteinuria): One of the early signs of CKD is the presence of protein in the urine, which indicates that the kidneys' filtering system is becoming damaged. Proteinuria can accelerate kidney damage if left untreated. ACE inhibitors and ARBs help reduce the amount of protein that leaks into the urine by lowering the pressure inside the kidneys, which improves the filtering process and protects kidney function.

- Slow the Progression of CKD: By reducing blood pressure and proteinuria, ACE inhibitors and ARBs help slow the progression of kidney damage. Research has shown that these medications can delay the need for dialysis or a kidney transplant in people with CKD, especially when taken early in the disease's course.

Who Should Take ACE Inhibitors or ARBs?

These medications are commonly prescribed for people with CKD who also have high blood pressure or diabetes, as these conditions put extra strain on the kidneys. Your healthcare provider may recommend starting one of these medications if:

- You have high blood pressure, particularly if it's difficult to control with other medications.
- You have diabetes, as blood sugar and blood pressure management are critical to protecting kidney health.
- You have been diagnosed with proteinuria, even if your blood pressure is normal. Reducing protein in the urine can help prevent further damage to your kidneys.

In some cases, people may be prescribed both an ACE inhibitor and an ARB, but this depends on individual health circumstances and should always be guided by your healthcare provider.

Potential Side Effects

While ACE inhibitors and ARBs are generally well-tolerated, they can have side effects. Some of the most common include:

- Cough (more common with ACE inhibitors)
- Elevated potassium levels (hyperkalemia), which can cause heart problems if not monitored
- Dizziness or lightheadedness, especially when first starting the medication
- Kidney function changes, which may require dose adjustments or close monitoring

It's important to regularly check blood pressure and kidney function while taking these medications. Your doctor may order periodic blood tests to monitor potassium levels and kidney health.

Working with Your Doctor

Your doctor will assess your overall health, kidney function, and risk factors to determine if an ACE inhibitor or ARB is appropriate for you. In some cases, adjustments to the dosage may be necessary based on how well your kidneys are functioning. Monitoring is key, so keeping up with regular appointments and blood tests will help ensure the medication is doing its job without causing complications.

Medications to Control Blood Pressure and Blood Sugar

For people with Chronic Kidney Disease (CKD), managing blood pressure and blood sugar levels is critical in slowing the progression of kidney damage. These two factors are closely linked with kidney health, and uncontrolled blood pressure or diabetes can significantly worsen CKD. Fortunately, there are medications available that specifically target these issues and help protect your kidneys.

1. Medications to Control Blood Pressure
Why Managing Blood Pressure is Important for CKD

High blood pressure (hypertension) is one of the leading causes of kidney damage and is a common complication of CKD. Elevated blood pressure increases the force with which blood flows through the kidneys, damaging the small blood vessels and filtering units (glomeruli). Over time, this leads to scarring, reduced kidney function, and eventually, kidney failure if left untreated. Keeping your blood pressure under control is essential to protecting your kidneys.

Common Medications for Controlling Blood Pressure in CKD

Several classes of medications are used to lower blood pressure in people with CKD. Your doctor will choose the most appropriate one based on your individual health needs. These medications include:

- ACE Inhibitors and ARBs: As discussed earlier, these are first-line treatments for managing high blood pressure in CKD patients. They not only lower blood pressure but also protect the kidneys by reducing proteinuria (protein leakage into the urine).
- Calcium Channel Blockers: These medications, such as amlodipine or diltiazem, help relax the blood vessels, making it easier for blood to flow and reducing blood pressure. Calcium channel blockers are often prescribed when ACE inhibitors or ARBs alone don't adequately control blood pressure.
- Diuretics (Water Pills): Diuretics, like furosemide or hydrochlorothiazide, help your body get rid of excess salt and water, which reduces the amount of fluid in your blood vessels. This lowers blood pressure and helps reduce swelling (edema), which is common in CKD patients.
- . Beta Blockers: Beta blockers, such as metoprolol or atenolol, reduce the workload on your heart by slowing the heart rate and lowering blood pressure. They are often used when CKD is accompanied by heart disease or high blood pressure that isn't controlled by other medications.
- Aldosterone Antagonists: Medications like spironolactone block the effects of aldosterone, a hormone that can raise blood pressure by increasing salt retention. These drugs can help lower blood pressure and reduce the risk of further kidney damage.

Monitoring Blood Pressure

Your doctor will work with you to establish a target blood pressure, typically below 130/80 mm Hg for people with CKD. Regular monitoring is crucial to ensure that your medications are effectively controlling your blood pressure without causing unwanted side effects. You may be asked to check your blood pressure at home, and adjustments to your medication regimen may be made based on the results.

2. Medications to Control Blood Sugar
Why Managing Blood Sugar is Important for CKD

Diabetes is one of the leading causes of CKD, as high blood sugar levels can damage the small blood vessels in the kidneys over time. Keeping your blood sugar under control is crucial to slowing the progression of kidney damage. For people with both CKD and diabetes, maintaining tight blood sugar control can significantly reduce the risk of kidney failure.

Common Medications for Controlling Blood Sugar in CKD

There are several classes of medications used to help manage blood sugar levels in people with diabetes. Some medications are safer for people with CKD than others, and your doctor will choose the best option based on your kidney function.

- **Insulin:** For many people with advanced CKD and diabetes, insulin is the preferred treatment because it can be adjusted based on blood sugar levels and doesn't rely on the kidneys for clearance. Insulin injections help regulate blood sugar levels, reducing the strain on the kidneys.
- **Metformin:** Metformin is often the first-line treatment for type 2 diabetes, but in people with CKD, it may be used with caution. While it's effective at lowering blood sugar, metformin can sometimes cause a buildup of lactic acid in the blood in people with severely reduced kidney function. Your

doctor may adjust the dose or switch to another medication if your kidney function declines.

- **SGLT2 Inhibitors:** Medications like empagliflozin and dapagliflozin are newer drugs that help the kidneys excrete excess glucose through urine. Studies have shown that SGLT2 inhibitors not only help control blood sugar but also protect kidney function by reducing the risk of CKD progression.
- **GLP-1 Receptor Agonists:** Drugs like liraglutide and semaglutide help control blood sugar by stimulating insulin release and reducing appetite. These medications have been shown to provide kidney protection and may help slow the progression of CKD in people with diabetes.
- **DPP-4 Inhibitors:** Medications like sitagliptin and linagliptin increase insulin production after meals and decrease the amount of glucose released by the liver. These drugs are often used in people with mild to moderate CKD because they don't stress the kidneys as much as other diabetes medications.

Monitoring Blood Sugar

For people with CKD and diabetes, regular blood sugar monitoring is essential. Your doctor will work with you to determine the appropriate target range for your blood sugar levels, and you'll likely need to check them frequently at home. Keeping your HbA1c (a measure of your average blood sugar over the past 2-3 months) in the recommended range, usually below 7%, is important to prevent further kidney damage.

Phosphate Binders and Other Supplements to Support Kidney Health

As Chronic Kidney Disease (CKD) progresses, the kidneys lose their ability to properly filter out waste products, including phosphorus. High phosphorus levels can lead to several complications, including bone and cardiovascular problems. To help manage this, healthcare providers often prescribe phosphate binders and recommend other supplements to support kidney health.

1. Phosphate Binders

Why Phosphate Binders Are Necessary

In CKD, the kidneys are unable to remove excess phosphorus from the blood. This leads to hyperphosphatemia, or elevated phosphorus levels, which can cause serious health issues such as:

- **Bone damage:** High phosphorus levels can lead to weakened bones, a condition known as renal osteodystrophy. When phosphorus levels rise, calcium is pulled from the bones, making them brittle and more prone to fractures.
- **Heart and blood vessel problems:** Excess phosphorus can cause calcium deposits to form in the blood vessels, heart, and lungs. This condition, known as vascular calcification, increases the risk of heart disease, stroke, and other cardiovascular complications.

To prevent these issues, phosphate binders are prescribed to help lower phosphorus levels in the blood. These medications work by binding to phosphorus in the food you eat, preventing it from being absorbed into the bloodstream and allowing it to be eliminated through the stool.

Types of Phosphate Binders

There are several different types of phosphate binders, each with its own benefits and potential side effects. Your doctor will choose the best option based on your needs and how well your body tolerates the medication.

- **Calcium-based binders:** These include calcium carbonate and calcium acetate, which bind to phosphorus in the gut. They are commonly prescribed and are effective at lowering phosphorus levels. However, taking too much calcium can lead to high blood calcium levels, which may cause calcification in blood vessels or increase the risk of kidney stones.
- **Non-calcium-based binders:** For patients who need to avoid excess calcium, non-calcium phosphate binders like sevelamer or lanthanum are often used. These medications are effective at lowering phosphorus levels without increasing calcium levels, reducing the risk of vascular calcification.
- **Iron-based binders:** Newer phosphate binders, such as ferric citrate and sucroferric oxyhydroxide, also bind to phosphorus in the gut and have the added benefit of boosting iron levels, which can help with anemia, another common issue in CKD patients.

How to Take Phosphate Binders

Phosphate binders are typically taken with meals to prevent phosphorus from being absorbed during digestion. It's important to follow your healthcare provider's instructions carefully, as the timing of these medications can impact their effectiveness. Additionally, you'll likely need to adhere to a low-phosphorus diet, avoiding foods like dairy products, processed foods, and certain meats, which are high in phosphorus.

2. Other Supplements to Support Kidney Health

In addition to phosphate binders, people with CKD may need other supplements to address specific nutrient deficiencies or manage complications associated with the disease. Here are some of the most commonly recommended supplements:

- **Vitamin D:** The kidneys play a crucial role in converting vitamin D into its active form, which helps regulate calcium and phosphorus levels in the body. As kidney function declines, this process becomes impaired, leading to vitamin D deficiency. Many CKD patients are prescribed active forms of vitamin D, such as calcitriol or paricalcitol, to help maintain bone health and balance calcium levels.

- **Calcium:** While excessive calcium can be harmful, some CKD patients may need calcium supplements to maintain healthy bones. This is particularly important for those who are using non-calcium-based phosphate binders, as they may not be getting enough calcium from other sources. However, calcium supplements should only be taken under a doctor's guidance to avoid complications.

- **Iron:** CKD often leads to anemia, a condition where the body doesn't produce enough red blood cells, resulting in fatigue and weakness. Iron supplements, either in oral or intravenous form, are commonly prescribed to boost iron levels and improve red blood cell production, particularly in patients who are also taking erythropoiesis-stimulating agents (ESAs).

- **Erythropoiesis-Stimulating Agents (ESAs):** ESAs, such as epoetin alfa or darbepoetin alfa, are medications used to treat anemia by stimulating the production of red blood cells. These are often used in conjunction with iron supplements to manage the anemia that comes with CKD.
- **Sodium Bicarbonate:** Some people with CKD develop metabolic acidosis, a condition in which the body's blood becomes too acidic due to poor kidney function. Sodium bicarbonate (baking soda) can be prescribed to neutralize the acid in the blood and help maintain a healthy pH balance.

3. Monitoring and Adjusting Supplement Use

Since supplements and phosphate binders can affect calcium, phosphorus, and other mineral levels in the body, it's essential to monitor these levels regularly. Your healthcare provider will order blood tests to check for imbalances and adjust your supplements or medications as needed. It's important not to take any over-the-counter supplements or vitamins without consulting your doctor, as some may interact with your prescribed medications or be harmful to your kidneys.

Managing Side Effects and Adjusting Medications

What to Expect When Taking Kidney-Related Medications

Taking medications for Chronic Kidney Disease (CKD) is a key part of managing the disease and slowing its progression. However, these medications can sometimes come with side effects and specific instructions that may affect your day-to-day routine. Understanding what to expect when taking kidney-related medications can help you stay prepared and manage your treatment effectively.

1. Common Side Effects

Many of the medications used to manage CKD—such as those for controlling blood pressure, reducing phosphorus levels, or managing anemia—can have side effects. While not everyone experiences them, it's important to know what to watch for and how to manage any discomfort.

- **ACE Inhibitors and ARBs:** These medications, used to control blood pressure and protect kidney function, can sometimes cause a dry cough (more common with ACE inhibitors), elevated potassium levels (hyperkalemia), and dizziness. Some people may experience a drop in blood pressure, leading to lightheadedness, especially when standing up quickly.

- **Diuretics:** Diuretics, or "water pills," can cause increased urination, which is expected as they help your body eliminate excess fluid. However, they can also lead to low potassium levels, dehydration, or muscle cramps. Some people might experience dizziness, especially when starting the medication or adjusting the dose.

- **Phosphate Binders:** Common side effects of phosphate binders include gastrointestinal issues, such as nausea, constipation, diarrhea, or bloating. Calcium-based phosphate binders may also increase the risk of elevated calcium levels, which can lead to other complications, such as kidney stones or vascular calcification.

- **Iron Supplements:** Oral iron supplements may cause gastrointestinal discomfort, including constipation, nausea, or a metallic taste in the mouth. Intravenous (IV) iron can sometimes cause allergic reactions or vein irritation, though this is rare.

- **Erythropoiesis-Stimulating Agents (ESAs):** ESAs, used to treat anemia, can sometimes cause flu-like symptoms, including joint or muscle pain, headaches, and fever. Some patients may also experience high blood pressure or blood clotting, which requires careful monitoring.

- **Sodium Bicarbonate:** If prescribed sodium bicarbonate for metabolic acidosis, some patients may experience bloating, gas, or increased thirst. Rarely, taking too much sodium bicarbonate can lead to electrolyte imbalances, so careful monitoring is important.

2. Adjusting to New Medications

When starting a new medication, your body may need time to adjust. It's common to experience mild side effects during the first few days or weeks of treatment, and these often improve over time. However, if you experience severe or persistent side effects, contact your healthcare provider. They may need to adjust the dose, switch to a different medication, or provide additional treatments to manage side effects.

It's also important to follow your medication instructions carefully. Some kidney-related medications must be taken with food, while others need to be taken on an empty stomach. Phosphate binders, for example, should always be taken with meals to be effective, while other medications may require specific timing to avoid interactions with other drugs or supplements.

3. Monitoring and Blood Tests

When taking medications for CKD, regular monitoring through blood tests is essential to ensure that the treatments are working as intended and that they are not causing harmful side effects. Your doctor will likely schedule routine lab work to check for:

- **Kidney function:** Blood tests, such as creatinine and GFR, will track how well your kidneys are filtering waste.
- **Electrolytes:** Medications like diuretics or ACE inhibitors can affect electrolyte levels, including potassium, sodium, and calcium. Regular monitoring ensures these levels stay within a healthy range.
- **Blood pressure:** Since many CKD medications impact blood pressure, your healthcare provider will regularly check it to ensure that it remains within target levels.
- **. Phosphorus and calcium levels:** Phosphate binders and supplements affect these levels, so frequent blood tests help ensure that phosphorus and calcium remain balanced to protect your bones and cardiovascular system.

- **Hemoglobin and iron levels:** For those taking iron supplements or ESAs, blood tests will monitor for anemia and ensure that your red blood cell count is stable.

Your doctor may also adjust your medications based on these test results, especially if you develop imbalances or complications.

4. Managing Multiple Medications

Many people with CKD are prescribed several medications to manage different aspects of their health, such as blood pressure, blood sugar, phosphorus levels, and anemia. Managing multiple medications can be challenging, but there are steps you can take to stay organized and avoid interactions:

- **Create a medication schedule:** Use a pill organizer or keep a written schedule to track when to take each medication. Some people find it helpful to set alarms or reminders on their phone.
- **Watch for interactions:** Certain medications or supplements can interact with each other, reducing their effectiveness or causing side effects. Always inform your healthcare provider and pharmacist about all the medications and supplements you're taking, including over-the-counter drugs, herbal remedies, and vitamins.
- **Take medications as prescribed:** Skipping doses or stopping medications without your doctor's approval can worsen your condition. If you're struggling with side effects or have concerns about your medications, talk to your doctor before making any changes.
- **Regular check-ins:** Keep up with your scheduled appointments and lab work to make sure that your medications are still appropriate and working well for you.

5. Potential Long-Term Effects

Some medications used in CKD treatment may have long-term effects, both positive and negative. For example, ACE inhibitors and ARBs provide long-term protection for your kidneys by controlling blood pressure and reducing proteinuria, but they may increase potassium levels over time. Diuretics can help manage fluid retention but may lead to electrolyte imbalances if used for extended periods.

Long-term use of certain supplements, like calcium-based phosphate binders, can increase the risk of complications like hypercalcemia (high calcium levels) or vascular calcification. Your healthcare provider will regularly assess whether these medications and supplements are still the best options for you and may switch to alternatives as needed.

6. Communicating with Your Doctor

It's essential to maintain open communication with your healthcare provider about how your medications are affecting you. Let them know if you experience any new or worsening symptoms, and ask questions about your treatment plan. Regular check-ins allow for adjustments and ensure that your medications are helping to manage CKD effectively.

Working with Your Doctor to Make Changes as Needed

Chronic Kidney Disease (CKD) is a dynamic condition, and your treatment plan will likely need to be adjusted over time as your health and kidney function change. Working closely with your doctor ensures that your medications, lifestyle choices, and treatment strategies remain effective and aligned with your evolving needs. Here's how you can collaborate with your healthcare team to make necessary changes:

1. Regular Checkups and Monitoring

Routine checkups and lab tests are essential in monitoring how well your treatment is working and determining if any adjustments are needed. These appointments allow your doctor to assess:

- **Kidney function:** Blood tests to measure creatinine, GFR, and other markers will show how well your kidneys are functioning. Changes in these values may indicate a need to adjust your medications.
- **Blood pressure:** Keeping your blood pressure within the target range is crucial for slowing CKD progression. If your blood pressure is consistently too high or low, your doctor may modify your treatment.
- **Electrolyte levels:** Medications like diuretics and phosphate binders can affect electrolyte balance, so your doctor will regularly monitor levels of potassium, calcium, and phosphorus. Adjustments may be needed to prevent complications.

- **Blood sugar levels:** If you have diabetes, managing your blood sugar is key to protecting your kidneys. Regular monitoring of your blood sugar levels helps your doctor determine if your current treatment is effective or if changes are necessary.

2. Addressing Side Effects

As you take medications for CKD, you may experience side effects that impact your daily life. If side effects become troublesome or affect your quality of life, it's important to discuss them with your healthcare provider. They may be able to:

- **Adjust the dosage:** Sometimes, side effects can be managed by lowering the dose of a medication. Your doctor may start you on a lower dose and gradually increase it, or reduce the dosage if side effects are severe.
- **Switch to a different medication:** If one medication is causing intolerable side effects, your doctor may suggest an alternative treatment. For example, if an ACE inhibitor causes a persistent cough, your doctor might switch you to an ARB.
- **Add another medication:** In some cases, adding a medication to counteract side effects may help. For example, if diuretics cause low potassium levels, your doctor might prescribe a potassium supplement.

Never stop taking your medications or change the dose on your own. Always consult your doctor first so they can guide you through safe and effective options for managing side effects.

3. Adjusting Medications as Kidney Function Changes

As CKD progresses, your kidney function may decline, which can affect how your body processes certain medications. Some medications may need to be reduced or stopped altogether to avoid causing further damage or complications.

- **Renal dosing:** Your doctor will adjust the dosage of your medications based on your kidney function, a process known as renal dosing. This is particularly important for medications that are filtered by the kidneys, such as antibiotics, pain relievers, or certain blood pressure medications.
- **Switching to safer alternatives:** As kidney function declines, some medications can become too risky to continue. Your doctor may switch you to alternative drugs that are less likely to strain the kidneys or cause harmful side effects.
- **Dialysis:** If you reach end-stage renal disease (Stage 5 CKD), dialysis may be required to filter waste from your blood. Your medication regimen will need to be carefully managed to ensure that drugs are not removed too quickly during dialysis and that any complications are minimized.

4. Keeping Track of Symptoms and Progress

Paying attention to changes in your body and symptoms is an important way to help your doctor make informed decisions about your treatment. Keep a journal of your symptoms, noting any:

- **New or worsening symptoms:** Let your doctor know if you experience symptoms like increased fatigue, swelling, changes in urination, or difficulty breathing. These could indicate a need for changes in your treatment.
- **Side effects:** Document any side effects from medications, such as nausea, dizziness, or muscle cramps, and share this information with your doctor.

- **Lifestyle changes:** If you've made dietary or exercise adjustments, track your progress and discuss it with your doctor. They can help you refine these changes to better support your kidney health.

5. Reviewing Your Medication List Regularly

Over time, your list of medications may grow as new treatments are added to address evolving health issues. Regularly reviewing your medication list with your doctor is important to:

- **Avoid medication overload:** Taking too many medications can increase the risk of side effects and drug interactions. Your doctor can help streamline your medication regimen, eliminating unnecessary drugs and reducing the risk of complications.
- **Check for interactions:** Some medications may interact with each other or with over-the-counter supplements. Reviewing your full list of medications, including vitamins and herbal supplements, helps your doctor catch potential interactions.
- **Update dosing:** As your health changes, your doctor may need to adjust the dosage of certain medications to ensure they remain effective and safe.

6. Seeking a Second Opinion

If you feel unsure about your treatment plan or are facing complex decisions about your kidney care, seeking a second opinion can provide valuable insight. Another healthcare provider may offer a different perspective on your condition or suggest alternative treatments. Always feel empowered to ask for a second opinion, especially if you're considering major treatments like dialysis or a kidney transplant.

7. Staying Informed About New Treatments

CKD research is constantly evolving, and new treatments are regularly being developed. Ask your doctor about any advances in CKD treatment that may be appropriate for your condition, including:

- **New medications:** Keep up to date with new drug options that may better manage your symptoms or slow the progression of CKD.

- **Clinical trials:** Your doctor can inform you if there are clinical trials available that offer access to experimental treatments or cutting-edge therapies.

CHAPTER FOUR

LIFESTYLE CHANGES TO SUPPORT KIDNEY HEALTH

The Role of Diet in Managing CKD

Low-Sodium, Low-Protein, and Kidney-Friendly Diets: What You Need to Know

Diet plays a crucial role in managing Chronic Kidney Disease (CKD). Making the right dietary choices can help slow the progression of CKD, protect kidney function, and improve your overall health. For people with CKD, following a kidney-friendly diet often means reducing sodium and protein intake, as well as carefully managing other nutrients like potassium and phosphorus. Let's break down what a kidney-friendly diet looks like and how these adjustments can support kidney health.

1. Low-Sodium Diet
Why Sodium Matters

Sodium is a mineral that helps balance fluids in the body, but when your kidneys are damaged, they have a harder time regulating sodium and fluid levels. Too much sodium can lead to fluid retention, increased blood pressure, and swelling (edema), all of which can strain your kidneys and worsen CKD. Lowering your sodium intake can help manage these symptoms and prevent further kidney damage.

Tips for Following a Low-Sodium Diet

- **Limit processed and packaged foods:** Many processed foods contain high amounts of sodium, even those that don't taste salty. This includes canned soups, frozen meals, snack foods, and deli meats. Whenever possible, opt for fresh, whole foods that you prepare at home.
- **Choose low-sodium alternatives**: Look for low-sodium or sodium-free versions of your favorite foods, such as soups, sauces, and snacks. Always read the labels to ensure you're choosing products with reduced sodium content.
- **Cook with herbs and spices instead of salt:** To add flavor to your meals without using salt, experiment with herbs, spices, lemon juice, or garlic. Many seasonings can enhance the taste of your food while keeping sodium intake low.
- **Rinse canned foods:** If you use canned vegetables or beans, rinse them under water to remove excess sodium before cooking.

For most people with CKD, the daily sodium intake should be limited to about 1,500 to 2,000 milligrams, but your doctor or dietitian will provide specific guidelines based on your health needs.

2. Low-Protein Diet
Why Protein Matters

Protein is an essential nutrient, but in CKD, too much protein can strain the kidneys. When your body breaks down protein, it produces waste products like urea, which the kidneys normally filter out. In people with CKD, damaged kidneys struggle to remove these waste products, which can lead to a buildup of toxins in the blood. Reducing your protein intake can ease the workload on your kidneys and help prevent further damage.

Tips for Following a Low-Protein Diet

- **Choose high-quality protein sources:** When you do consume protein, focus on high-quality sources like lean meats, poultry, fish, eggs, and plant-based proteins like tofu or legumes. High-quality protein provides essential amino acids while producing less waste for the kidneys to filter.
- **Work with a dietitian:** Because your protein needs will depend on your stage of CKD, it's important to work with a healthcare provider or dietitian who can help you determine the right amount of protein for your condition. Typically, the recommended protein intake for CKD patients is about 0.6 to 0.8 grams of protein per kilogram of body weight per day, but this varies based on individual health factors.
- **Limit portion sizes:** Pay attention to portion sizes of protein-rich foods. You can still enjoy meat, fish, or eggs, but in smaller quantities to reduce the strain on your kidneys.

Reducing protein intake doesn't mean eliminating it completely. It's about finding a balance that meets your nutritional needs while protecting your kidneys.

3. Kidney-Friendly Diets: Managing Potassium and Phosphorus

In addition to limiting sodium and protein, people with CKD often need to monitor their intake of potassium and phosphorus. Both of these minerals can accumulate in the blood when kidney function is impaired, leading to complications.

Potassium

Potassium helps regulate heart function and muscle contractions, but high levels can be dangerous for people with CKD. Hyperkalemia (high potassium) can cause irregular heartbeats and other serious problems. To manage potassium levels, it's important to limit or avoid foods that are high in potassium, including:

- Bananas
- Oranges and orange juice
- Potatoes
- Tomatoes
- Spinach
- Avocados

Instead, focus on low-potassium alternatives, such as apples, berries, grapes, and green beans. Your doctor or dietitian can guide you on the right amount of potassium for your diet based on your blood test results.

Phosphorus

Phosphorus is another mineral that people with CKD need to monitor closely. When phosphorus builds up in the blood, it

can lead to weakened bones and calcification of the blood vessels and organs. Many processed and packaged foods contain added phosphorus, so it's important to avoid foods high in phosphorus, such as:
- Dairy products (milk, cheese, yogurt)
- Nuts and seeds
- Dark colas and soft drinks
- Processed meats and fast foods

Instead, opt for phosphorus-friendly options like non-dairy milk (almond or rice milk), fresh fruits, and vegetables. If you're unable to control phosphorus levels through diet alone, your doctor may prescribe phosphate binders to help remove excess phosphorus from your bloodstream.

4. Hydration: The Role of Fluids in a Kidney-Friendly Diet

Proper hydration is important for kidney health, but in CKD, fluid management can be tricky. As kidney function declines, the body may retain excess fluids, leading to swelling, high blood pressure, and shortness of breath. Depending on your stage of CKD, your doctor may recommend limiting your fluid intake to prevent fluid overload.

- Monitor fluid intake: Keep track of how much water and other fluids (like soups, tea, and juice) you drink each day. Your doctor will give you a target amount based on your kidney function.
- . Avoid overhydration: While it's important to stay hydrated, drinking too much water can lead to complications if your kidneys aren't able to process it effectively. Stick to your recommended fluid limits.

- Watch for signs of fluid retention: If you notice swelling in your legs, feet, or hands, or if you experience shortness of breath, these could be signs of fluid retention. Let your doctor know if these symptoms appear.

Foods to Avoid and Foods to Include to Protect Your Kidneys

For people with Chronic Kidney Disease (CKD), choosing the right foods can make a significant difference in protecting kidney function and overall health. Certain foods can increase the strain on your kidneys or worsen complications like high blood pressure, high potassium, or phosphorus levels. On the other hand, some foods can help maintain a healthy balance of nutrients and support kidney function. Here's a guide to foods you should avoid and those you should include in a kidney-friendly diet.

Foods to Avoid
When managing CKD, it's important to limit or avoid foods that can negatively impact kidney function or lead to imbalances in key nutrients like sodium, potassium, and phosphorus.

1. High-Sodium Foods As mentioned earlier, sodium can cause fluid retention and raise blood pressure, which puts extra strain on the kidneys. It's important to minimize your intake of high-sodium foods, including:
• Processed and packaged foods: Items like chips, crackers, canned soups, frozen meals, and ready-made sauces often contain large amounts of sodium.

- Fast food and takeout: Many restaurant meals, especially fast food, are high in sodium. Avoiding or limiting these foods can help keep your sodium intake in check.
- Pickled and cured foods: Foods like pickles, olives, sauerkraut, and cured meats (such as bacon, ham, and sausages) are typically high in sodium due to the brining or curing process.
- Salty snacks: Potato chips, pretzels, and other salty snacks should be avoided, as they can quickly add up to your daily sodium limit.

2. High-Potassium Foods High levels of potassium can be dangerous for people with CKD, especially as kidney function declines. Certain fruits and vegetables are naturally high in potassium and should be limited or avoided, including:
- . Bananas
- Oranges and orange juice
- Potatoes (including sweet potatoes)
- Tomatoes (including tomato sauce)
- Avocados
- Spinach
- Mushrooms

Instead, opt for lower-potassium alternatives such as apples, berries, grapes, lettuce, cucumbers, and carrots.

3. High-Phosphorus Foods Excess phosphorus can weaken your bones and cause other complications in CKD. Many processed foods and drinks have added phosphorus, and some naturally phosphorus-rich foods should be avoided or limited:

- **Dairy products:** Milk, cheese, yogurt, and ice cream are high in phosphorus.
- **Nuts and seeds:** These foods are rich in phosphorus, so they should be eaten sparingly.
- **Cola and dark sodas:** Many dark colas contain added phosphorus, so it's best to avoid these beverages.
- **Processed meats:** Items like hot dogs, sausages, and deli meats often contain added phosphorus in the form of preservatives.

4. High-Protein Foods (in moderation) While protein is essential for your body, too much of it can place a burden on your kidneys. Foods high in protein that should be limited include:
- Red meats (beef, pork, lamb)
- Poultry with skin
- High-fat dairy products
- Large portions of fish or eggs

Your healthcare provider or dietitian will help you determine how much protein you need based on your stage of CKD, but moderation is key to preventing overburdening your kidneys.

Foods to Include

While CKD often requires limiting certain foods, there are still many nutritious options that can help support kidney health without placing additional strain on your kidneys.

1. Low-Sodium Alternatives To reduce your sodium intake while still enjoying flavorful meals, focus on:

- **Fresh fruits and vegetables:** These are naturally low in sodium. Opt for fresh or frozen produce rather than canned, and rinse canned vegetables if you do use them.
- **Herbs and spices:** Use herbs like basil, oregano, parsley, and spices like garlic powder, paprika, or lemon juice to flavor your meals without adding salt.
- **Whole grains:** Choose low-sodium, whole-grain options like plain oatmeal, quinoa, or whole-grain bread with minimal added salt.

2. Low-Potassium Foods Many fruits and vegetables are low in potassium and can be enjoyed regularly, such as:

- Apples, berries (strawberries, blueberries, raspberries), grapes, and pears
- Cabbage, cauliflower, lettuce, and bell peppers
- Green beans, cucumbers, and carrots
- . Pineapple and watermelon (in moderation)

These low-potassium options can help you maintain a healthy, balanced diet without risking high potassium levels.

3. Low-Phosphorus Foods For people with CKD, it's important to choose foods that are low in phosphorus, such as:

- Non-dairy milk substitutes: Almond milk, rice milk, and other plant-based milk alternatives are typically lower in phosphorus than dairy milk.
- Fresh fruits and vegetables: Most fruits and vegetables are naturally low in phosphorus, making them great choices for a kidney-friendly diet.

- Lean meats and poultry: Opt for small portions of lean meats, like skinless chicken or turkey, in moderation. Choose fresh cuts over processed meats.

4. Healthy Fats Healthy fats are an important part of any diet, including one designed for CKD. These fats can help provide energy without straining your kidneys:
- Olive oil: A heart-healthy source of monounsaturated fat that can be used in cooking or drizzling on salads.
- Avocado oil: Though avocados are high in potassium, avocado oil is a kidney-friendly fat option.
- Flaxseed oil: Rich in omega-3 fatty acids, flaxseed oil can support heart health and help reduce inflammation, which is important for people with CKD.

5. Protein Sources (in moderation) It's important to eat enough high-quality protein to meet your nutritional needs without overloading your kidneys. Choose lean or plant-based sources of protein:

- Small portions of chicken or turkey (without skin): These lean meats are good sources of protein and are lower in fat compared to red meats.
- Fish (in moderation): Fatty fish like salmon or trout can be enjoyed in small portions, as they are high in omega-3 fatty acids, which support heart and kidney health.
- Tofu and beans (in moderation): Plant-based protein sources are great for kidney health, but they should be eaten in smaller portions to avoid excess protein intake.

The Importance of Staying Hydrated

Staying properly hydrated is important for everyone, but it becomes especially crucial for individuals with Chronic Kidney Disease (CKD). Water helps the kidneys function by flushing out waste and keeping the body's balance of fluids and electrolytes stable. However, in people with CKD, hydration requires careful management to avoid complications, such as fluid overload or dehydration. Understanding how much water you should drink and when can help you support your kidney health.

Why Hydration Matters for Kidney Health
The kidneys play a central role in regulating the body's fluid levels. They filter excess water, waste, and toxins from the blood, which are then excreted in the urine. When your kidneys are functioning properly, staying hydrated helps this filtration process run smoothly.
For people with CKD, the kidneys struggle to maintain this balance as their function declines. In some cases, the kidneys may not filter out enough fluid, leading to fluid retention, while in others, too much water can lead to further strain on already weakened kidneys. Finding the right hydration balance is key to managing CKD and preventing complications.

How Much Water Should You Drink?
The amount of water you should drink depends on your stage of CKD, your overall health, and any other conditions you

may have. For some people with early-stage CKD, staying well-hydrated can help support kidney function. For those with more advanced stages, limiting fluid intake may be necessary to avoid fluid overload, which can lead to swelling, high blood pressure, or difficulty breathing.

Here are some general guidelines, but it's essential to work with your doctor to determine the right amount for you:

- **Early-Stage CKD (Stages 1-2):** In the early stages of CKD, staying hydrated can help the kidneys continue to flush out waste effectively. Drinking enough water is typically encouraged unless there are other medical conditions, such as heart failure, that require limiting fluids. The general recommendation is to drink around 8 cups (2 liters) of water a day, though your individual needs may vary.
- **Later-Stage CKD (Stages 3-5):** As kidney function declines in later stages, fluid retention becomes a concern. Your doctor may recommend limiting your fluid intake to avoid swelling (edema), high blood pressure, or fluid buildup in the lungs. In these cases, your fluid allowance may be reduced to a specific amount, such as 4-6 cups (1-1.5 liters) of water per day, including water from food and other beverages.

Signs of Fluid Overload and Dehydration

It's important to monitor your hydration levels to avoid both fluid overload and dehydration. Knowing the signs of each can help you make adjustments as needed.

Signs of Fluid Overload

If your kidneys aren't filtering out enough fluid, it can build up in your body, leading to:

- Swelling in the legs, ankles, feet, or hands (edema)
- Shortness of breath or difficulty breathing, especially when lying down
- Increased blood pressure
- Rapid weight gain due to fluid retention

If you experience any of these symptoms, contact your healthcare provider. They may recommend adjusting your fluid intake or modifying your medications to help manage the symptoms.

Signs of Dehydration

On the other hand, if you don't drink enough water, your kidneys may have a harder time filtering waste, leading to dehydration. Signs of dehydration include:

- Dark yellow urine or a strong odor
- Dry mouth or dry skin
- Dizziness or lightheadedness
- Feeling unusually thirsty
- Fatigue or lack of energy

If you notice signs of dehydration, it's important to increase your fluid intake gradually and let your doctor know. They can help guide you on how to rehydrate safely without overburdening your kidneys.

Tips for Managing Hydration with CKD

Balancing hydration while managing CKD can be challenging, but the following tips can help you stay on track:

- Monitor your fluid intake: If your doctor recommends limiting fluids, keep track of how much water you drink each day, including water from soups, coffee, tea, and other beverages. Measuring your intake helps ensure you stay within your recommended limit.

- Spread out your fluid intake: To avoid overwhelming your kidneys with too much fluid at once, try spreading out your water intake throughout the day. Take small sips rather than drinking large amounts at one time.
- Be mindful of foods with high water content: Fruits and vegetables like watermelon, cucumbers, and lettuce contain a lot of water and can contribute to your total fluid intake. If you're on fluid restrictions, factor in these foods when calculating your daily intake.
- Monitor your weight daily: Sudden weight gain can be a sign of fluid retention. Weigh yourself at the same time each day, and report any unexplained increases to your doctor.
- Limit salt intake: Eating too much sodium can make you thirsty and increase fluid retention. Reducing your sodium intake can help prevent these issues and make it easier to manage your fluid balance.
- Consider ice chips or frozen treats: If you're limiting fluids but feel thirsty, ice chips or small servings of frozen fruit can help quench your thirst without taking in too much water.

Exercise and Physical Activity

How Exercise Can Help Protect Your Kidneys

Exercise is an important part of a healthy lifestyle, and for people with Chronic Kidney Disease (CKD), it can provide several benefits that support kidney health and overall well-being. Regular physical activity helps manage some of the underlying conditions that contribute to kidney damage, such as high blood pressure, diabetes, and obesity. It also improves cardiovascular health, strengthens muscles, and boosts energy levels. While exercise won't reverse kidney damage, it can slow the progression of CKD and help you maintain a higher quality of life.

1. Managing Blood Pressure

High blood pressure is both a cause and a complication of CKD. When blood pressure is too high, it puts extra strain on the kidneys, which can accelerate kidney damage. Exercise is a proven way to lower blood pressure naturally. Here's how it helps:

- **Improved heart function:** Regular aerobic exercise strengthens the heart, allowing it to pump blood more efficiently. This reduces the pressure on blood vessels and lowers overall blood pressure.
- **Reduced vascular resistance:** Exercise helps keep blood vessels flexible and healthy, which reduces the resistance against blood flow. This, in turn, helps lower blood pressure.

- **Weight management:** Maintaining a healthy weight through exercise can help reduce blood pressure, as excess weight is a risk factor for hypertension.

By keeping your blood pressure in check, you can protect your kidneys from further damage.

2. Controlling Blood Sugar Levels

For people with diabetes, managing blood sugar is critical to preventing kidney damage. Exercise helps lower blood sugar by increasing insulin sensitivity, allowing your muscles to use glucose (sugar) more effectively. Regular physical activity can:

- **Lower blood glucose levels:** During exercise, muscles take up glucose from the bloodstream for energy, which helps reduce blood sugar levels.
- **Improve insulin sensitivity:** After exercise, your body becomes more sensitive to insulin, meaning it can use insulin more effectively to regulate blood sugar. This is particularly beneficial for people with type 2 diabetes, as it helps keep blood sugar levels under control.

By managing blood sugar through exercise, you can help prevent or slow the progression of diabetic kidney disease.

3. Supporting Weight Management

Obesity is a significant risk factor for CKD and can worsen kidney damage by contributing to high blood pressure, diabetes, and cardiovascular disease. Regular physical activity helps with weight management by:

- **Burning calories:** Aerobic activities like walking, cycling, or swimming help burn calories, which supports weight loss or maintenance.

- **Boosting metabolism:** Building muscle through strength training can increase your resting metabolic rate, meaning you burn more calories even when you're not exercising.
- **Reducing fat around the abdomen:** Abdominal fat is particularly harmful to kidney health, as it is associated with higher risks of diabetes and hypertension. Exercise helps reduce visceral fat, which can improve overall kidney health. Maintaining a healthy weight through regular exercise reduces the strain on your kidneys and supports better overall health.

4. Improving Cardiovascular Health

People with CKD are at higher risk for cardiovascular diseases, such as heart disease and stroke. Exercise helps strengthen the cardiovascular system by:

- **Improving circulation:** Regular aerobic exercise improves blood flow, which is important for heart health and reduces the risk of heart-related complications.
- **Lowering cholesterol levels:** Exercise can help lower LDL (bad) cholesterol and raise HDL (good) cholesterol, which supports healthier blood vessels and reduces the risk of cardiovascular disease.
- **Reducing inflammation:** Chronic inflammation can harm blood vessels and the kidneys, but regular physical activity helps lower inflammation markers, supporting both heart and kidney health.

By improving heart health, you reduce the risk of cardiovascular complications that are common in CKD patients and can protect your kidneys from further damage.

5. Enhancing Mental Health and Well-Being

Living with CKD can be physically and emotionally challenging, often leading to feelings of stress, anxiety, or depression. Exercise is known to boost mental health by:

- **Releasing endorphins:** Physical activity stimulates the release of endorphins, which are natural chemicals in the brain that promote feelings of well-being and reduce stress.
- **Improving sleep:** Regular exercise can help regulate sleep patterns, which is important for both physical and mental health.
- **Reducing anxiety and depression:** Exercise has been shown to reduce symptoms of anxiety and depression, which can help improve your overall quality of life when managing a chronic condition like CKD.

By enhancing your mental and emotional well-being, exercise can help you stay motivated and positive as you manage your kidney disease.

6. Strengthening Muscles and Reducing Fatigue

People with CKD often experience muscle weakness and fatigue, especially as kidney function declines. Exercise can help combat these issues by:

- **Building muscle strength:** Strength-training exercises, such as lifting light weights or using resistance bands, can help build and maintain muscle mass, which is often lost in CKD patients.
- **Boosting energy levels:** Regular physical activity increases your overall stamina and reduces fatigue, making it easier to perform daily tasks and stay active.

- **Improving balance and flexibility:** Exercises like yoga or tai chi can improve balance and flexibility, which can help prevent falls and enhance overall mobility.

By strengthening muscles and reducing fatigue, exercise can improve your physical resilience and help you maintain an active lifestyle.

Finding the Right Balance Between Activity and Rest

When managing Chronic Kidney Disease (CKD), it's important to strike a balance between staying active and getting enough rest. Exercise is beneficial for your overall health, but it's also crucial to listen to your body and avoid overexertion. Finding this balance can help you maintain physical strength, mental well-being, and protect your kidney health without causing unnecessary fatigue or strain on your body.

1. Understanding Your Energy Levels

People with CKD often experience fatigue, particularly as the disease progresses. This can be caused by several factors, including anemia (a lack of red blood cells), poor nutrition, and the body's inability to filter toxins effectively. Exercise can help boost energy levels, but overdoing it may lead to exhaustion or worsen symptoms like muscle aches or shortness of breath.

To avoid pushing yourself too hard, it's essential to:

- **Listen to your body:** Pay attention to how you feel before, during, and after physical activity. If you start to feel overly tired or experience pain, dizziness, or shortness of breath, it's time to rest.
- **Set realistic goals:** Start slow and gradually increase your activity levels. For example, begin with short walks or light stretching and gradually build up to longer or more challenging exercises over time.

- **Keep a log:** Track your daily energy levels, activities, and rest periods in a journal. This will help you see patterns and understand when you need more rest or can handle more activity.

2. Incorporating Rest and Recovery

Rest is just as important as exercise when it comes to managing CKD. Adequate rest allows your body to recover from physical activity, repair muscle tissue, and restore energy levels. Some ways to ensure you're getting enough rest include:

- **Prioritize sleep:** Aim for 7-9 hours of sleep each night. A regular sleep routine can improve energy levels and reduce the feelings of fatigue associated with CKD. If sleep is a challenge, talk to your doctor about ways to improve sleep quality.
- **Take breaks:** During the day, give yourself time to rest between activities. If you're feeling fatigued after exercising, rest for a bit before continuing with your day.
- **Use relaxation techniques:** Practices such as meditation, deep breathing, or gentle yoga can help your body relax and recover. These techniques can also reduce stress, which is important for overall kidney health.

3. Customizing Your Activity Routine

Everyone's energy levels and physical capabilities are different, especially when dealing with a chronic condition like CKD. It's important to customize your activity routine to fit your needs and health goals. Here are a few tips to help:

- **Talk to your healthcare provider:** Before starting any new exercise routine, consult with your doctor or a physical therapist who can recommend appropriate activities based on your stage of CKD, overall health, and physical abilities.

- **Combine light exercise with rest:** On days when you feel more fatigued, opt for light activities like stretching or walking rather than more strenuous workouts. Balance these activities with periods of rest to avoid overexertion.
- **Alternate between activities:** Vary your physical activities to avoid working the same muscles day after day. For example, alternate between walking, strength training, and yoga to give different parts of your body time to rest and recover.

4. Knowing When to Rest

While it's important to stay active, there are times when rest should take priority. Knowing when to take a break can prevent you from overworking your body and allow for better long-term management of CKD. You should prioritize rest if you experience:

- **Excessive fatigue:** If you feel unusually tired, even after a good night's sleep or after light physical activity, it may be a sign that your body needs more rest.
- **Pain or discomfort:** Muscle soreness after exercise is normal, but if you experience persistent pain, it's important to rest and let your body heal before resuming activity.
- **Shortness of breath or chest pain:** These are signs that your body is under strain and may need immediate rest. If these symptoms occur, stop exercising and consult your doctor.
- **Dizziness or lightheadedness:** If you feel faint or unsteady during or after physical activity, it's a sign that your body may need more rest.

5. Adjusting Your Routine Over Time

As your CKD progresses, your energy levels and physical abilities may change. It's important to adjust your exercise routine accordingly to ensure you're still getting the benefits of physical activity without overburdening your body. You may need to:

- **Reduce the intensity of your workouts:** As your CKD advances, you may find it helpful to switch to low-impact activities like swimming, cycling, or gentle yoga.
- **Shorten the duration of exercise sessions:** Instead of aiming for longer workouts, try shorter, more frequent bursts of activity. For example, you could do 10-15 minutes of light exercise several times a day instead of a single 30-minute session.
- **Incorporate more rest days:** As your kidney disease progresses, you may need to take more frequent rest days to allow your body time to recover. Listen to your body and give it the rest it needs.

Tips for Staying Active Without Overdoing It

Staying physically active is an essential part of managing Chronic Kidney Disease (CKD), but it's important to pace yourself to avoid overexertion. Balancing activity with rest ensures you reap the benefits of exercise without putting unnecessary strain on your body. Here are some practical tips to help you stay active while protecting your kidneys and maintaining your energy levels.

1. Start Slowly and Gradually Increase Activity
When starting a new exercise routine, it's important to ease into it, especially if you haven't been very active. Jumping into strenuous workouts can lead to injury or fatigue, so focus on building up your strength and endurance gradually.

- **Begin with low-impact activities:** Walking, swimming, or cycling are great low-impact exercises that are gentle on the joints and kidneys while still providing cardiovascular benefits. Start with short sessions (10-15 minutes) and gradually increase the duration as you become more comfortable.
- **Increase intensity over time:** Once your body adjusts to regular exercise, you can slowly increase the intensity. For example, add light resistance training or increase the pace of your walks, but avoid pushing yourself too hard too quickly.

2. Break Up Exercise Into Short Sessions
If long workout sessions feel overwhelming or leave you too fatigued, try breaking your exercise into smaller, more

manageable chunks throughout the day. This allows you to stay active without exhausting yourself.

- **Mini-workouts:** Instead of aiming for one 30-minute session, try doing three 10-minute sessions spread throughout the day. These shorter bursts of activity are easier to fit into your routine and provide the same health benefits as longer workouts.
- **Active breaks:** Incorporate small amounts of movement during your day, such as taking a short walk during lunch breaks or doing gentle stretches while watching TV. These small actions add up and help you stay active without overdoing it.

3. Listen to Your Body

It's important to stay in tune with how your body feels before, during, and after exercise. While regular physical activity is beneficial, pushing through pain, discomfort, or extreme fatigue can lead to setbacks.

- **Stop if you feel pain:** Exercise shouldn't be painful. If you experience sharp pain, especially in your muscles or joints, stop and rest. Consult your healthcare provider if the pain persists.
- **Rest when needed:** Feeling unusually tired or lightheaded during or after exercise may be a sign that you need to rest. It's okay to take breaks or scale back your exercise routine on days when your energy is low.
- **Monitor your breathing:** Pay attention to your breathing during exercise. If you find it hard to catch your breath, slow down or take a break. You should be able to maintain a conversation during low-intensity exercise without gasping for air.

4. Set Realistic Goals

Setting achievable exercise goals can help keep you motivated without overexerting yourself. Focus on what you can do and build from there, gradually increasing your activity level as your strength and stamina improve.

- **Make small, attainable goals:** Instead of aiming for big milestones, set smaller, more manageable goals. For example, start by walking for 10 minutes a day, and slowly increase to 15 or 20 minutes over time.
- **Celebrate progress:** Acknowledge the small victories, such as walking an extra block or adding a few more repetitions to your strength training. Celebrating these achievements can boost your confidence and keep you motivated.

5. Incorporate Strength and Flexibility Exercises

In addition to cardiovascular exercise, strength training and flexibility exercises can help maintain muscle mass, improve balance, and reduce the risk of injury.

- **Strength training:** Include light strength-training exercises, such as using resistance bands or lifting light weights. These exercises can be done 2-3 times a week to help build and maintain muscle. Be mindful of your form to avoid injury, and focus on controlled movements.
- **Stretching and flexibility:** Incorporating gentle stretching or yoga can improve your flexibility and balance. Stretching before and after exercise can help prevent stiffness and keep your muscles flexible.

6. Choose Activities You Enjoy
Staying active is easier and more sustainable when you engage in activities that you enjoy. Doing something you love can make exercise feel less like a chore and more like a fun part of your day.
- **Find activities that motivate you:** Whether it's dancing, gardening, swimming, or taking nature walks, choose activities that you genuinely enjoy. This will make it easier to stick to a regular routine and keep moving.
- **Make it social:** Exercising with a friend, family member, or group can make it more enjoyable and provide accountability. Walking with a friend or joining a fitness class can also boost motivation.

7. Stay Hydrated, But Don't Overdo It
It's important to stay hydrated during exercise, but if you have CKD, managing your fluid intake can be tricky. Your doctor may recommend limiting fluids to prevent fluid overload, so it's important to balance hydration carefully.
- **Sip water throughout the day:** Instead of drinking large amounts of water all at once, sip small amounts throughout the day to stay hydrated without overwhelming your kidneys.
- **Monitor your thirst:** If you're feeling thirsty during exercise, it's okay to drink small amounts of water. However, avoid drinking more than your recommended daily fluid intake.

8. Rest and Recover

Just as important as exercise is taking time to rest and recover. This allows your muscles to heal and prevents burnout or injury.

- **Schedule rest days:** Include rest days in your exercise routine to give your body time to recover. On rest days, you can still engage in gentle activities like stretching or walking, but avoid intense workouts.
- **Get adequate sleep:** Restful sleep is crucial for muscle recovery and overall energy levels. Aim for 7-9 hours of sleep each night to support your physical and mental well-being.

Reducing Stress

How Stress Affects Kidney Function
Stress is a normal part of life, but chronic or unmanaged stress can have a significant impact on your health, especially for people living with Chronic Kidney Disease (CKD). While stress itself doesn't cause CKD, it can contribute to complications that worsen kidney function. Understanding how stress affects your body and kidneys can help you take proactive steps to manage it and protect your health.

1. The Body's Response to Stress
When you experience stress, your body activates the "fight-or-flight" response, which releases hormones like cortisol and adrenaline. These hormones prepare your body to deal with a perceived threat by raising your heart rate, increasing blood pressure, and sending more blood to your muscles. While this response is helpful in short bursts, chronic stress keeps your body in this heightened state, which can lead to several health issues.

For people with CKD, chronic stress can worsen existing problems such as high blood pressure and inflammation, both of which directly affect kidney function. Over time, the negative effects of stress can contribute to the progression of kidney disease and increase the risk of cardiovascular complications.

2. Stress and High Blood Pressure

One of the most significant ways stress impacts kidney health is by contributing to high blood pressure (hypertension). Chronic stress causes your blood vessels to tighten and increases your heart rate, which raises your blood pressure. For people with CKD, managing blood pressure is crucial, as high blood pressure can damage the small blood vessels in the kidneys, reducing their ability to filter waste from the blood.

- **Stress-induced hypertension:** Prolonged stress can lead to sustained high blood pressure, which accelerates kidney damage. If stress goes unaddressed, it can make it harder to control blood pressure, even with medication.
- **Impact on kidney function:** High blood pressure increases the pressure on the kidneys' delicate filtering units (glomeruli), causing damage over time. This can lead to a decline in kidney function and may worsen CKD.

3. Stress, Cortisol, and Inflammation

Cortisol is a hormone released by the adrenal glands in response to stress. While cortisol helps the body manage short-term stress, long-term elevated levels of cortisol can lead to inflammation. Chronic inflammation has been linked to worsening kidney function in people with CKD.

- **Inflammation and kidney health:** Chronic inflammation can damage the blood vessels and tissues in the kidneys, leading to scarring (fibrosis) and impaired kidney function. For people with CKD, managing inflammation is key to slowing the progression of the disease.
- **Stress and the immune system:** Prolonged stress weakens the immune system, making the body more susceptible to

infections and illnesses, which can further strain the kidneys and other organs.

4. Stress and Unhealthy Coping Mechanisms

In addition to the direct physical effects of stress, it can also lead to unhealthy behaviors that negatively impact kidney health. People experiencing chronic stress may turn to coping mechanisms like overeating, smoking, or drinking alcohol, which can exacerbate CKD symptoms.

- **Unhealthy diet choices:** Stress often leads to emotional eating, particularly of high-sodium, high-fat, or sugary foods, which can contribute to weight gain, high blood pressure, and increased cholesterol—all of which strain the kidneys.
- **Smoking and alcohol:** Some people may turn to smoking or alcohol to cope with stress. Both smoking and excessive alcohol use can raise blood pressure, reduce blood flow to the kidneys, and worsen kidney damage.
- **Lack of physical activity:** Stress can also lead to a lack of motivation to exercise, which is vital for managing CKD. Physical inactivity can worsen conditions like high blood pressure, diabetes, and obesity, all of which affect kidney function.

5. Stress and Sleep Disturbances

Chronic stress can disrupt your sleep patterns, making it harder to get the restful sleep your body needs. Poor sleep can have a direct impact on kidney function by increasing inflammation, raising blood pressure, and contributing to insulin resistance, which is particularly harmful for people with diabetes and CKD.

- **Sleep and kidney health:** Studies have shown that poor sleep quality and short sleep duration are associated with a faster decline in kidney function. Getting enough sleep is crucial for allowing the body to repair and recover, especially for people managing CKD.

6. The Mental Health Connection

Living with a chronic illness like CKD can contribute to feelings of stress, anxiety, or depression. Mental health challenges, if left unaddressed, can further complicate the management of CKD. Stress and anxiety may make it harder to follow treatment plans, take medications regularly, or adhere to a kidney-friendly diet.

- **Anxiety and depression:** People with CKD may feel overwhelmed by the management of their condition, leading to anxiety or depression. Mental health struggles can make it difficult to stay motivated, engage in self-care, or keep up with medical appointments.
- **The impact on kidney health:** Poor mental health has been linked to worse outcomes in people with CKD. Depression, in particular, has been shown to accelerate the progression of kidney disease, making it important to seek mental health support when needed.

Simple Relaxation Techniques: Meditation, Deep Breathing, and Mindfulness

Managing stress is essential for people with Chronic Kidney Disease (CKD), as prolonged stress can negatively affect kidney function. Incorporating simple relaxation techniques such as meditation, deep breathing, and mindfulness into your daily routine can help lower stress levels, reduce blood pressure, and improve your overall well-being. These techniques are easy to practice and can be done almost anywhere, making them a valuable tool for maintaining balance and reducing the negative effects of stress on your kidneys.

1. Meditation

Meditation is a relaxation technique that involves focusing your attention and calming your mind. It has been shown to reduce stress, improve emotional health, and lower blood pressure—key benefits for people managing CKD.

- **How to Practice Meditation:** Find a quiet, comfortable place to sit or lie down. Close your eyes and take deep breaths, focusing on each inhalation and exhalation. If your mind starts to wander, gently bring your attention back to your breath. Start with just 5-10 minutes a day, gradually increasing the time as you become more comfortable with the practice.

- **Benefits of Meditation:** Regular meditation can help reduce cortisol levels, lower blood pressure, and decrease feelings of anxiety or depression. By calming the mind and body, meditation promotes relaxation and helps mitigate the negative effects of chronic stress.

- **Types of Meditation:** There are many forms of meditation, including guided meditation (where someone leads you through the practice), mantra meditation (where you silently repeat a word or phrase), and body scan meditation (where you focus on different parts of your body to relax them). Experiment with different styles to find what works best for you.

2. Deep Breathing Exercises

Deep breathing exercises are one of the simplest and most effective ways to reduce stress. When you're stressed, your breathing becomes shallow, which can contribute to feelings of anxiety and tension. Deep breathing helps calm the nervous system, reduce blood pressure, and promote a sense of relaxation.

- **How to Practice Deep Breathing:** Sit or lie down in a comfortable position. Place one hand on your chest and the other on your abdomen. Take a slow, deep breath in through your nose, allowing your abdomen to rise as your lungs fill with air. Then, slowly exhale through your mouth, feeling your abdomen fall. Repeat this process for 5-10 minutes, focusing on your breath and allowing any tension in your body to release.
- **Benefits of Deep Breathing:** Deep breathing helps activate the body's relaxation response, reducing cortisol levels and calming the mind. It can also help improve oxygen flow throughout your body, which can promote better overall health.

- **Tips for Consistency:** Deep breathing exercises can be done anytime you feel stressed or anxious. Whether you're at home, at work, or in a waiting room, taking a few moments to focus on your breath can help lower your stress levels and restore a sense of calm.

3. Mindfulness

Mindfulness is the practice of being fully present in the moment, without judgment or distraction. It encourages you to observe your thoughts, feelings, and physical sensations without becoming overwhelmed by them. Mindfulness is particularly helpful for managing stress because it shifts your focus away from worries about the past or future and grounds you in the present.

- **How to Practice Mindfulness:** Start by focusing on your breath, as you would in meditation. Then, gradually expand your awareness to include your surroundings, such as the sounds you hear, the sensations in your body, and your emotions. The key is to observe without judgment—simply notice what you're experiencing without trying to change it or become consumed by it.
- **Benefits of Mindfulness:** Practicing mindfulness can help you become more aware of your body's signals, allowing you to better manage stress, pain, and emotional challenges. Over time, mindfulness can reduce anxiety, improve emotional resilience, and help you feel more in control of your mental and physical well-being.
- **Mindful Activities:** Mindfulness can be practiced during everyday activities, such as eating, walking, or even washing dishes. Focus on the sensations and details of the activity, such as the taste of food or the feeling of water on your

hands. By engaging fully in the moment, you can cultivate mindfulness throughout the day.

4. Progressive Muscle Relaxation

Progressive muscle relaxation (PMR) is a technique that involves tensing and then relaxing different muscle groups in the body. This practice helps release physical tension and promotes a deep state of relaxation.

- **How to Practice PMR:** Start by sitting or lying down in a comfortable position. Begin with your feet and gradually work your way up through your body, tensing each muscle group for a few seconds, then slowly releasing the tension. Focus on the contrast between the tension and the relaxation in each muscle group. By the end of the exercise, your body should feel more relaxed and calm.
- **Benefits of PMR:** PMR helps reduce physical tension that builds up in response to stress. It also promotes awareness of where tension is held in the body, helping you release it more effectively in the future.

5. Yoga and Tai Chi

Yoga and tai chi are mind-body practices that combine physical movement, breathing exercises, and meditation. Both practices are known for their stress-reducing benefits and can help improve flexibility, balance, and mental clarity.

- **Yoga:** Yoga involves gentle stretching and postures that promote relaxation and mindfulness. Many yoga practices include deep breathing and meditation, making it a holistic approach to stress reduction. Even a short daily yoga routine can help release tension, improve circulation, and enhance your sense of well-being.

- **Tai Chi:** Tai chi is a form of martial arts that involves slow, flowing movements and deep breathing. It's often described as "meditation in motion" and is especially helpful for improving balance, flexibility, and relaxation. Like yoga, tai chi is low-impact and can be practiced by people of all fitness levels.

CHAPTER FIVE

NATURAL REMEDIES AND ALTERNATIVE THERAPIES

Herbs and Supplements for Kidney Health

Natural Remedies That Support Kidney Function: Turmeric, Omega-3s, and More

In managing Chronic Kidney Disease (CKD), many people explore natural remedies alongside their medical treatments to support kidney function and overall health. While these natural options can't cure CKD, certain herbs, supplements, and foods have properties that may help reduce inflammation, support the body's immune response, and protect against further damage. Turmeric, omega-3 fatty acids, and other natural remedies are some of the most commonly used options.

1. Turmeric

Turmeric is a bright yellow spice commonly used in cooking, particularly in Indian cuisine. Its active ingredient, curcumin, has powerful anti-inflammatory and antioxidant properties, making it a popular natural remedy for a variety of health conditions, including CKD.

- **Anti-inflammatory properties:** Chronic inflammation is a key factor in the progression of CKD, and turmeric's ability to reduce inflammation can help protect the kidneys from further damage. By lowering inflammation in the body, curcumin may help slow the progression of kidney disease and reduce symptoms related to inflammation, such as pain or swelling.

- **Antioxidant effects:** Curcumin also acts as an antioxidant, which means it helps neutralize harmful free radicals that can damage cells and tissues, including those in the kidneys. This protection can support overall kidney health.

How to use turmeric: Turmeric can be added to food, such as soups, curries, or smoothies. It's also available as a supplement in capsule form, but it's important to consult your healthcare provider before taking turmeric supplements, especially if you are on blood-thinning medications, as turmeric can increase the risk of bleeding.

2. Omega-3 Fatty Acids

Omega-3 fatty acids, found in fish oil and certain plant oils, are known for their anti-inflammatory properties and heart health benefits. These essential fatty acids can help reduce inflammation in the kidneys and support overall cardiovascular health, which is crucial for people with CKD.

- **Reducing inflammation:** Omega-3 fatty acids, particularly EPA (eicosapentaenoic acid) and DHA (docosahexaenoic acid), have been shown to lower markers of inflammation in the body. Since inflammation plays a significant role in kidney damage, consuming omega-3s may help slow the progression of CKD and improve kidney function.

- **Heart health benefits:** People with CKD are at a higher risk of cardiovascular disease, and omega-3 fatty acids are known to reduce triglycerides, lower blood pressure, and support heart health. By improving cardiovascular health, omega-3s indirectly benefit kidney function as well.

Sources of omega-3s: Fatty fish like salmon, mackerel, and sardines are rich sources of omega-3s. Plant-based sources include flaxseeds, chia seeds, and walnuts. Fish oil supplements are also widely available, but it's important to check with your doctor before starting supplements, especially if you are taking blood-thinning medications.

3. Ginger

Ginger is another natural remedy known for its anti-inflammatory and antioxidant properties. It has been used for centuries to help with digestion, reduce nausea, and fight inflammation.

- **Anti-inflammatory effects:** Like turmeric, ginger contains compounds that help reduce inflammation in the body. This can be beneficial for people with CKD, as chronic inflammation can lead to kidney damage.

- **Improving digestion:** Ginger is also known for its ability to improve digestion and reduce nausea, which can be helpful for people with CKD who experience digestive issues related to their condition or medications.

How to use ginger: Fresh ginger can be added to teas, smoothies, or meals. It's also available in supplement form, but as with any supplement, it's important to consult your doctor before starting ginger supplements, especially if you are on medication for blood pressure or blood thinning.

4. Garlic

Garlic is another popular natural remedy with potential benefits for kidney health. It has antioxidant, anti-inflammatory, and blood pressure-lowering properties.

- **Lowering blood pressure:** Garlic is known to help lower blood pressure, which is especially important for people with CKD, as high blood pressure is a major contributor to kidney damage.

- **Antioxidant and anti-inflammatory properties:** The compounds in garlic, such as allicin, act as antioxidants, helping to neutralize free radicals and reduce inflammation, both of which can benefit kidney health.

How to use garlic: Fresh garlic can be used in cooking, or you can take garlic supplements. As with other supplements, consult your healthcare provider before taking garlic in supplement form, as it can interact with medications.

5. Green Tea

Green tea is rich in antioxidants called catechins, which have been shown to reduce inflammation and protect cells from oxidative damage.

- **Antioxidant effects:** The catechins in green tea help protect kidney cells from damage caused by free radicals, which can slow the progression of CKD.

- **Heart health:** Green tea is also known for its benefits in supporting heart health, which is important for CKD patients who are at a higher risk of cardiovascular disease.

How to use green tea: Drinking 1-2 cups of green tea a day can provide antioxidant benefits. However, green tea contains caffeine, so it's important to monitor your intake if you're sensitive to caffeine or have been advised to limit it.

6. Cranberry

Cranberry is well-known for its benefits in urinary tract health, particularly in preventing urinary tract infections (UTIs). People with CKD are more prone to UTIs, which can worsen kidney function if left untreated.

- **Preventing UTIs:** Cranberries contain compounds that prevent bacteria from adhering to the walls of the urinary tract, reducing the risk of infection.

- **Supporting kidney health:** By preventing UTIs, cranberry products may help protect the kidneys from further damage caused by infections.

How to use cranberry: Cranberry juice or supplements can be consumed, but it's important to choose low-sugar options, as high sugar intake can negatively affect kidney health, particularly for those with diabetes.

7. Dandelion Root

Dandelion root is commonly used as a natural diuretic, which helps the body get rid of excess water and sodium. This can be particularly beneficial for people with CKD who experience fluid retention.

- **Natural diuretic:** Dandelion root encourages the kidneys to excrete excess fluid, which can help reduce swelling (edema) and lower blood pressure.

- **Supporting liver and kidney health:** Dandelion root is also thought to support liver health, which can indirectly benefit the kidneys by helping detoxify the body.

How to use dandelion root: Dandelion root can be consumed as a tea or in supplement form. However, people with CKD should use dandelion with caution, as too much can disrupt electrolyte balance. Always consult your doctor before using diuretics, including natural ones.

The Role of Antioxidants in Fighting Inflammation

Antioxidants play a crucial role in protecting the body from oxidative stress, which can lead to chronic inflammation and damage to cells, including those in the kidneys. For people with Chronic Kidney Disease (CKD), managing inflammation is particularly important, as it contributes to the progression of the disease. By including antioxidant-rich foods and supplements in your diet, you may help reduce oxidative damage and support kidney health.

1. Understanding Oxidative Stress and Inflammation

Oxidative stress occurs when there is an imbalance between free radicals (unstable molecules that can damage cells) and the body's ability to neutralize them with antioxidants. Free radicals are produced naturally in the body during processes like metabolism, but they can also result from exposure to pollutants, toxins, or unhealthy lifestyle choices such as smoking and a poor diet.

When free radicals build up in the body, they can cause damage to proteins, lipids, and DNA, leading to inflammation. Chronic inflammation is a key factor in the development and progression of many diseases, including CKD.

Antioxidants are substances that help neutralize free radicals and protect the body from oxidative damage. They can be found in a variety of foods, especially fruits, vegetables, and certain herbs. By fighting oxidative stress, antioxidants help reduce inflammation, which is critical for slowing the progression of kidney disease.

2. Antioxidant-Rich Foods for Kidney Health

Incorporating antioxidant-rich foods into your diet can provide protection against oxidative stress and inflammation. Here are some foods that are particularly high in antioxidants and supportive of kidney health:

- **Berries:** Blueberries, strawberries, raspberries, and blackberries are packed with antioxidants, including vitamin C and flavonoids. Berries are also low in potassium, making them a great choice for people with CKD who need to manage their potassium intake.

- **Leafy greens:** Spinach, kale, and collard greens are rich in vitamins A, C, and K, as well as antioxidants like lutein and zeaxanthin. These vegetables help protect cells from oxidative damage. However, for individuals with advanced CKD, it's important to monitor potassium levels, as some greens can be high in potassium.

- **Red grapes:** Red grapes contain powerful antioxidants, including resveratrol, which has been shown to reduce inflammation and protect against oxidative stress. Grapes are also low in potassium, making them a kidney-friendly fruit option.

- **Apples:** Apples are high in fiber and vitamin C, and their antioxidant content helps fight inflammation. Apples are also low in potassium, making them a safe choice for people with CKD.

- **Garlic and onions:** Both garlic and onions contain sulfur compounds and flavonoids that have antioxidant and anti-inflammatory effects. They can be added to meals for flavor and health benefits without adding sodium, which is important for managing CKD.

- **Cabbage:** Cabbage is rich in vitamin C and other antioxidants. It's low in potassium and can be included in a kidney-friendly diet. The antioxidants in cabbage help protect the kidneys from oxidative damage.

- **Bell peppers:** Red, yellow, and orange bell peppers are high in vitamin C and antioxidants like beta-carotene, which help reduce inflammation. Bell peppers are low in potassium, making them a suitable vegetable for people with CKD.

- **Cranberries:** In addition to supporting urinary tract health, cranberries are high in antioxidants, including vitamin C and polyphenols, which can help reduce oxidative stress.

3. Antioxidant Supplements

While it's best to get antioxidants from whole foods, supplements can also be beneficial in certain cases. Some common antioxidant supplements that may support kidney health include:

- **Vitamin C:** Vitamin C is a powerful antioxidant that helps protect cells from oxidative damage. However, people with CKD should be cautious with vitamin C supplements, as high doses can lead to the formation of oxalate, which can cause kidney stones. Always consult your doctor before taking vitamin C supplements.

- **Vitamin E:** Vitamin E is another potent antioxidant that protects cell membranes from oxidative damage. Some studies have suggested that vitamin E supplements may help reduce inflammation in CKD patients. However, it's important to follow your doctor's recommendations regarding supplementation.

- **Coenzyme Q10 (CoQ10):** CoQ10 is a naturally occurring antioxidant that plays a role in energy production and reducing oxidative stress. Some studies have shown that CoQ10 supplementation may help improve kidney function and reduce inflammation in people with CKD. Consult your healthcare provider before starting a CoQ10 supplement.

- **Alpha-lipoic acid:** Alpha-lipoic acid is an antioxidant that helps regenerate other antioxidants, such as vitamins C and E. It has been studied for its potential to reduce oxidative stress and improve kidney function in people with diabetes and CKD. Always check with your healthcare provider before adding this supplement to your routine.

- **Resveratrol:** Found naturally in red grapes and red wine, resveratrol is known for its antioxidant and anti-inflammatory effects. While the research on resveratrol supplementation for CKD is still in the early stages, it may offer protective benefits. However, it's important to talk to your doctor before taking resveratrol supplements, especially if you are on other medications.

4. How Antioxidants Help Reduce Inflammation

Antioxidants work by neutralizing free radicals and preventing them from damaging cells. This, in turn, reduces the body's inflammatory response, which is triggered when free radicals cause oxidative damage.

For people with CKD, inflammation is a major factor in the progression of the disease. By incorporating antioxidants into your diet or taking supplements under medical supervision, you can help reduce this inflammation, protect kidney cells, and slow the progression of kidney damage.

5. Combining Antioxidants with Medical Treatment

While antioxidants can be a helpful addition to your diet, they should not replace medical treatments prescribed by your doctor. It's important to view antioxidant-rich foods and supplements as complementary to your medical treatment plan, rather than as a cure or standalone solution.

Before adding any new supplements to your routine, always consult your healthcare provider to ensure they don't interfere with your current medications or treatments. Some supplements, even those with antioxidant properties, can interact with blood thinners, blood pressure medications, or other drugs commonly prescribed to CKD patients.

How to Safely Use Herbal Supplements Alongside Medications

For people managing Chronic Kidney Disease (CKD), it's common to explore herbal supplements as a way to complement traditional treatments. However, combining herbal remedies with prescribed medications requires careful consideration to ensure safety and avoid negative interactions. While some herbs and supplements may offer benefits for kidney health, they can also interact with medications or have unwanted side effects if not used properly. It's crucial to consult your healthcare provider before incorporating any new herbal treatments into your routine.

1. The Importance of Consulting with Your Healthcare Provider

Before starting any herbal supplements, it's essential to talk to your doctor, particularly if you are already taking prescribed medications for CKD or related conditions such as high blood pressure, diabetes, or heart disease. Here's why this is important:

- **Avoiding drug interactions:** Herbal supplements can interact with prescription medications, potentially making them less effective or increasing the risk of side effects. For example, some herbs may increase the effects of blood thinners, leading to excessive bleeding, or they may raise blood pressure, complicating CKD management.

- **Ensuring proper dosing:** Herbal supplements, like medications, should be taken at the correct dose to avoid toxicity or adverse effects. Your doctor can help determine whether an herbal supplement is safe for you and guide you on the appropriate dosage.

- **Monitoring kidney function:** Many herbal supplements are processed by the kidneys, and taking too much of certain herbs can overburden your kidneys or worsen CKD. Regular monitoring of your kidney function is essential when using any supplements to ensure they are not causing harm.

2. Herbs to Use with Caution

Some herbs and natural remedies, though commonly used, may pose risks for people with CKD if taken in large amounts or without medical supervision. Here are a few herbs to be cautious of:

- **St. John's Wort:** This herb is often used to treat depression or anxiety, but it can interfere with many prescription medications, including those for high blood pressure and diabetes. St. John's Wort can also affect how your body metabolizes medications, making them less effective.

- **Ginkgo Biloba:** Ginkgo is used to improve memory and circulation, but it can increase the risk of bleeding, especially if you're taking blood-thinning medications. People with CKD should be particularly cautious, as ginkgo can also affect blood flow to the kidneys.

- **Licorice Root:** While licorice root is sometimes used for digestive issues and respiratory infections, it can raise blood pressure and cause fluid retention—both of which are harmful for people with CKD. Excessive licorice intake can also lead to electrolyte imbalances, which can further strain the kidneys.

- **Echinacea:** Echinacea is commonly taken to boost the immune system and fight colds, but it may increase inflammation in people with autoimmune conditions or those prone to allergies. For people with CKD, who may already have impaired immune function, it's important to be cautious with immune-stimulating herbs.

- **Horsetail:** Horsetail is often used as a diuretic, but it can lead to a loss of potassium, which can cause electrolyte imbalances. For people with CKD, managing potassium levels is crucial, so horsetail should be used only under strict medical guidance.

3. Herbs That May Support Kidney Health

While some herbs require caution, others may offer potential benefits for kidney health when used correctly. Here are a few herbs that may complement traditional CKD treatments, but always under your doctor's supervision:

- **Turmeric:** As mentioned earlier, turmeric's active compound, curcumin, has anti-inflammatory and antioxidant properties. When used in moderation, turmeric may help reduce inflammation in the kidneys, but it's important to discuss appropriate dosage with your healthcare provider.

- **Astragalus:** Astragalus is a traditional Chinese herb used to support immune function and reduce inflammation. Some studies suggest it may help protect kidney function, but it should only be taken with your doctor's approval, as it can interact with certain medications.

- **Dandelion Root:** Dandelion root is used as a natural diuretic, helping the body eliminate excess fluid. It may be helpful for managing fluid retention in people with CKD, but it can also affect electrolyte levels, so careful monitoring is needed.

- **Ginger:** Ginger has anti-inflammatory properties and can help alleviate nausea, which may be a side effect of certain CKD medications. However, ginger can also thin the blood, so consult your doctor if you are taking blood thinners or have a bleeding disorder.

4. Potential Interactions Between Supplements and CKD Medications

When using herbal supplements alongside CKD medications, it's important to be aware of potential interactions. Some common types of medications prescribed for CKD may interact with herbal remedies:

- **Blood pressure medications:** Many herbs can either raise or lower blood pressure, which may interfere with medications aimed at controlling hypertension. For example, herbs like licorice root can increase blood pressure, while others like garlic or hawthorn can lower it too much, especially if taken in large amounts.

- **Blood thinners (anticoagulants):** Herbs like ginkgo biloba, garlic, ginger, and turmeric can thin the blood, increasing the risk of bleeding if taken with anticoagulant medications like warfarin. It's essential to monitor blood clotting factors if using these herbs.

- **Diuretics:** Many herbs have diuretic properties, which can lead to excessive fluid loss and electrolyte imbalances when taken with prescribed diuretics. Dandelion root, horsetail, and green tea are examples of natural diuretics that should be used cautiously.

- **Diabetes medications:** Some herbal supplements, such as ginseng or fenugreek, can lower blood sugar levels. When taken alongside diabetes medications, this can lead to hypoglycemia (dangerously low blood sugar levels).

5. Tips for Safely Using Herbal Supplements

Here are some general guidelines for safely incorporating herbal supplements into your CKD management plan:

• **Talk to your doctor:** Always consult with your healthcare provider before starting any herbal supplements, especially if you are taking prescription medications. Your doctor can help you assess the safety of the supplement and guide you on the proper dosage.

• **Choose reputable brands:** Not all supplements are created equal. Look for high-quality, reputable brands that provide clear labeling and have been tested for purity and safety. Avoid products with undisclosed ingredients or exaggerated claims.

• **Start with small doses:** If your doctor approves the use of an herbal supplement, start with a low dose and monitor your body's response. This approach helps you avoid potential side effects or interactions.

• **Keep track of side effects:** Monitor your body for any adverse reactions, such as changes in blood pressure, digestive issues, or signs of fluid retention. Report any side effects to your doctor immediately.

• **Regularly review your medication list:** Keep an updated list of all medications, supplements, and herbs you are taking, and share it with your healthcare provider. This helps prevent dangerous interactions and ensures your treatment plan is optimized for your health.

Acupuncture and Massage Therapy

How Complementary Therapies Can Improve Blood Flow and Reduce Stress

Complementary therapies, such as acupuncture, massage therapy, and yoga, have become increasingly popular for managing various health conditions, including Chronic Kidney Disease (CKD). While these therapies are not substitutes for medical treatment, they can play a supportive role in improving blood flow, reducing stress, and enhancing overall well-being. By promoting relaxation and better circulation, complementary therapies can help alleviate some of the symptoms associated with CKD and reduce the impact of stress on the kidneys.

1. Acupuncture

Acupuncture is a traditional Chinese medicine practice that involves inserting thin needles into specific points on the body to stimulate energy flow and promote healing. It has been used for thousands of years to treat various ailments and is believed to help restore balance in the body.

- **Improving blood flow:** Acupuncture has been shown to increase blood circulation by stimulating the release of certain chemicals in the body, including nitric oxide, which helps dilate blood vessels and improve blood flow. For people with CKD, improved blood circulation can support overall kidney function and reduce symptoms like swelling and poor circulation.

- **Reducing stress:** Acupuncture is known for its ability to reduce stress and anxiety. By stimulating the nervous system, it promotes the release of endorphins, the body's natural "feel-good" chemicals, which can help reduce the negative effects of chronic stress on the kidneys. Lowering stress levels can help manage high blood pressure, one of the major contributors to kidney damage in CKD.

- **Managing symptoms:** Acupuncture has been used to manage various symptoms associated with CKD, such as nausea, pain, and fatigue. For people undergoing dialysis, acupuncture may help reduce side effects like muscle cramps and itching, though more research is needed in this area.

How to incorporate acupuncture: Always work with a licensed and experienced acupuncturist, particularly one familiar with CKD. Acupuncture can be used alongside conventional treatments but should not replace any medical interventions prescribed by your doctor.

2. Massage Therapy

Massage therapy is another complementary therapy that has been shown to improve blood circulation, reduce stress, and enhance relaxation. Different types of massage, such as Swedish, deep tissue, and lymphatic drainage massage, can target specific needs depending on your symptoms.

- **Improving circulation:** Massage therapy helps improve blood flow by stimulating the soft tissues and muscles. This can be especially beneficial for people with CKD, who may experience poor circulation, particularly in the extremities. Better blood flow can help reduce swelling (edema) and alleviate muscle pain or tension.

- **Reducing stress and anxiety:** One of the most immediate benefits of massage therapy is its ability to reduce stress. Physical touch and gentle manipulation of the muscles promote relaxation and reduce the production of stress hormones like cortisol. By lowering stress levels, massage therapy can help prevent stress-related increases in blood pressure, which is critical for managing CKD.

- **Alleviating pain:** Massage can help relieve muscle pain and tension that may result from CKD or dialysis treatments. Regular massage therapy sessions can improve muscle flexibility and reduce the discomfort that often accompanies CKD.

How to incorporate massage therapy: Always consult your healthcare provider before starting massage therapy, especially if you have CKD, as certain types of massage (such as deep tissue) may not be suitable for people with advanced kidney disease. It's also important to work with a certified massage therapist who understands your condition and can tailor the massage to meet your specific needs.

3. Yoga

Yoga is a mind-body practice that combines physical postures, breathing exercises, and meditation to promote relaxation, improve flexibility, and enhance overall health. For people with CKD, yoga can provide both physical and mental benefits that support kidney function and improve quality of life.

- **Improving blood flow and circulation:** Many yoga poses encourage gentle stretching and movement, which can help improve blood flow throughout the body. This improved circulation can support heart health, lower blood pressure, and reduce swelling—key concerns for people with CKD.

- **Reducing stress and promoting relaxation:** Yoga is well-known for its stress-reducing effects. By incorporating deep breathing and mindfulness techniques, yoga helps calm the nervous system and lower stress hormone levels. Practicing yoga regularly can help reduce the impact of chronic stress on your kidneys, supporting better blood pressure control and overall kidney health.

- **Strengthening muscles and improving flexibility:** Yoga helps build strength and flexibility, which can improve mobility and reduce muscle stiffness. This can be particularly beneficial for people with CKD who experience fatigue or weakness due to their condition. By improving physical strength and endurance, yoga can help you stay more active and manage CKD symptoms more effectively.

How to incorporate yoga: Start with gentle or restorative yoga classes, particularly those designed for beginners or people with chronic conditions. Always check with your healthcare provider before starting a yoga routine, and work with an experienced instructor who understands the limitations of CKD.

4. Tai Chi

Tai Chi is a low-impact exercise that originated in China as a martial art and is now practiced worldwide for its health benefits. Tai Chi involves slow, flowing movements that promote balance, flexibility, and relaxation.

- **Improving circulation:** The gentle movements of Tai Chi help improve blood flow without putting too much strain on the body. Better circulation can benefit the kidneys by ensuring they receive enough oxygen and nutrients to function properly.

- **Reducing stress:** Like yoga, Tai Chi is often described as "meditation in motion." The focus on deep breathing and slow, controlled movements helps reduce stress and anxiety, which can have a positive effect on blood pressure and kidney function.

- **Supporting balance and mobility:** Tai Chi improves coordination, balance, and strength, which can help people with CKD stay physically active without risking injury. This form of exercise is gentle enough for people of all fitness levels and can be particularly beneficial for older adults or those with limited mobility.

How to incorporate Tai Chi: Tai Chi classes are often offered at community centers, health clubs, or through online programs. Start with a beginner class and consult with your healthcare provider before starting, particularly if you have any mobility issues or concerns related to CKD.

5. Breathing Exercises and Meditation

Breathing exercises and meditation are powerful tools for managing stress and promoting relaxation. They help calm the mind, reduce blood pressure, and improve circulation, all of which can benefit people with CKD.

- **Deep breathing for relaxation:** Deep breathing exercises, such as diaphragmatic breathing, encourage full oxygen exchange, which improves circulation and helps calm the nervous system. Practicing deep breathing regularly can reduce stress, lower blood pressure, and support overall well-being.

- **Meditation for stress relief:** Meditation is a practice that involves focusing your attention on the present moment. Whether it's through guided meditation, mindfulness, or body scan techniques, meditation helps reduce stress and anxiety, which is beneficial for managing CKD.

How to incorporate breathing exercises and meditation: Start with 5-10 minutes of deep breathing or meditation each day. Find a quiet space to sit or lie down, and focus on your breath or a calming thought. Gradually increase the duration as you become more comfortable with the practice.

The Benefits of Using Alternative Therapies with Medical Treatment

For individuals managing Chronic Kidney Disease (CKD), traditional medical treatments are the cornerstone of care. However, integrating alternative therapies alongside these treatments can provide additional benefits, helping to improve quality of life, reduce symptoms, and support overall kidney health. While these therapies should not replace conventional medicine, they can complement it by addressing symptoms like stress, pain, and fatigue, which are commonly associated with CKD.

1. Enhancing the Effectiveness of Medical Treatment

Alternative therapies can help improve the effectiveness of medical treatment by addressing underlying issues that can interfere with your body's ability to respond to conventional care. For example:

- **Improving circulation:** Practices such as yoga, Tai Chi, and acupuncture can improve blood flow, which may enhance the delivery of oxygen and nutrients to the kidneys and other vital organs. This can help your body respond better to medications and treatments prescribed by your doctor.

- **Reducing side effects:** Alternative therapies like acupuncture and massage can help reduce the side effects of medical treatments, such as muscle pain, fatigue, and nausea. For people undergoing dialysis, these therapies may provide relief from symptoms like muscle cramps, headaches, or stress.

- **Supporting mental and emotional health:** Chronic stress and emotional strain can make it more difficult for your body to heal and respond to treatment. Practices like meditation, mindfulness, and deep breathing exercises can reduce stress, improve mood, and promote a sense of calm, which can support the healing process.

2. Managing Symptoms Naturally

While medications are effective at treating many aspects of CKD, they may not address every symptom or discomfort associated with the condition. Integrating alternative therapies can provide a natural way to manage these symptoms, improving your overall well-being. Some common symptoms that alternative therapies can help manage include:

- **Chronic pain:** Chronic pain, particularly in the back or joints, is common in CKD. Massage therapy, acupuncture, and yoga can all help reduce pain naturally by improving circulation, reducing muscle tension, and promoting relaxation.

- **Fatigue:** Many people with CKD experience persistent fatigue, which can be difficult to manage with medications alone. Gentle physical activities like yoga or Tai Chi, along with mindfulness techniques, can help boost energy levels and combat fatigue.

- **Nausea:** For individuals undergoing dialysis or taking certain medications, nausea can be a common side effect. Acupuncture and ginger supplements have been shown to help alleviate nausea, providing a natural complement to traditional treatments.

3. Reducing Stress and Anxiety

Chronic stress and anxiety can have a negative impact on kidney health by contributing to high blood pressure, inflammation, and poor sleep. Alternative therapies such as meditation, deep breathing exercises, and acupuncture are proven stress-relievers that can help support mental and physical health.

- **Stress management:** Practices like meditation, mindfulness, and yoga are designed to calm the mind and reduce the body's production of stress hormones, such as cortisol. Lowering stress levels is critical for people with CKD, as chronic stress can exacerbate kidney damage and contribute to other complications, such as high blood pressure.

- **Improving mental health:** Dealing with CKD can take an emotional toll, leading to feelings of anxiety or depression. Incorporating complementary therapies like acupuncture, mindfulness, or breathing exercises can provide relief and help improve mood, making it easier to cope with the challenges of living with CKD.

4. Supporting Overall Wellness

Alternative therapies often focus on holistic wellness, addressing the body, mind, and spirit. For people with CKD, maintaining a sense of balance and well-being is essential for managing the disease long-term. Some benefits of using alternative therapies alongside medical treatment include:

- **Promoting relaxation and sleep:** Relaxation techniques like progressive muscle relaxation, meditation, and acupuncture can improve sleep quality, which is crucial for overall health and recovery. Better sleep helps reduce fatigue, stress, and blood pressure—all of which are important for managing CKD.

- **. Improving flexibility and strength:** Gentle exercises like yoga and Tai Chi promote physical strength, flexibility, and balance. These activities not only help you stay active but also reduce the risk of falls, injuries, and stiffness, which can result from inactivity or muscle weakness due to CKD.

- **Encouraging self-care and mindfulness:** Many alternative therapies promote mindfulness and self-awareness, helping individuals become more in tune with their bodies and health. This awareness can lead to better self-care habits, such as adhering to a healthy diet, staying active, and managing stress, which are all important for supporting kidney health.

5. Personalizing Your Care

One of the key benefits of using alternative therapies is the ability to tailor treatments to your individual needs and preferences. CKD affects people differently, and what works for one person may not work for another. Alternative therapies offer a range of options, allowing you to choose the methods that best suit your lifestyle and health goals.

- **Customizing your approach:** For example, if you prefer a more active way to reduce stress, yoga or Tai Chi might be a better fit. If you're looking for a passive method to reduce pain or anxiety, acupuncture or massage therapy may be more suitable. The ability to personalize your care makes it easier to integrate alternative therapies into your overall treatment plan.

- **Involving your healthcare provider:** To safely integrate alternative therapies, it's important to work with your healthcare provider to ensure that your chosen therapies complement, rather than interfere with, your medical treatment. Your doctor can help guide you on how to safely incorporate these therapies into your routine, adjusting your care plan as needed.

6. Combining Therapies for a Holistic Approach

By combining conventional medical treatments with alternative therapies, you can take a more holistic approach to managing CKD. This integrative approach addresses the physical, mental, and emotional aspects of the disease, promoting overall health and well-being.

- **Medical treatment:** Your doctor will likely prescribe medications to manage symptoms such as high blood pressure, fluid retention, or anemia. In more advanced stages of CKD, treatments like dialysis or even a kidney transplant may be necessary.

- **Complementary therapies:** Alongside these medical treatments, alternative therapies such as acupuncture, massage, yoga, and meditation can help manage symptoms, reduce stress, and improve your quality of life. Together, these approaches form a comprehensive treatment plan that supports your overall health.

CHAPTER SIX

MANAGING COMMON COMPLICATIONS OF CKD

High Blood Pressure

Why Blood Pressure Management is Crucial for Kidney Health

Managing blood pressure is one of the most critical aspects of caring for Chronic Kidney Disease (CKD). High blood pressure, also known as hypertension, is both a cause and a consequence of CKD. When left uncontrolled, high blood pressure can accelerate kidney damage, making the progression of the disease faster and more severe. Conversely, CKD can contribute to hypertension, creating a vicious cycle that puts both the kidneys and the cardiovascular system under strain. Let's explore why blood pressure management is crucial for protecting kidney health and slowing the progression of CKD.

How High Blood Pressure Damages the Kidneys

High blood pressure forces the heart to pump blood with greater force, increasing the pressure within the arteries and blood vessels throughout the body, including the kidneys. This constant pressure can damage the delicate filtering units of the kidneys, called nephrons, which are responsible for removing waste and excess fluids from the blood.

• **Damage to blood vessels:** Over time, the increased pressure damages the small blood vessels in the kidneys, reducing their ability to filter waste and regulate essential functions like fluid balance and blood pressure. The damage leads to scarring (fibrosis) within the kidneys, further impairing kidney function.

• **Worsening of CKD:** As kidney function declines due to hypertension, the kidneys become less effective at regulating blood pressure, leading to a cycle of increasing blood pressure and worsening kidney damage. This can result in faster progression to end-stage kidney disease (ESKD), requiring dialysis or a kidney transplant.

• **Development of proteinuria:** High blood pressure can also cause the kidneys to leak protein into the urine, a condition known as proteinuria. Proteinuria is both a sign of kidney damage and a risk factor for further decline in kidney function. Managing blood pressure is essential to prevent or reduce proteinuria and protect kidney health.

The Link Between CKD and Hypertension

CKD and hypertension are closely related. Not only can high blood pressure cause kidney damage, but impaired kidney function can also lead to high blood pressure. The kidneys play a key role in regulating blood pressure by controlling the balance of fluids and salts in the body. When the kidneys are damaged, they struggle to maintain this balance, leading to fluid retention and increased blood pressure.

• **Fluid retention:** As kidney function declines, the kidneys are less able to remove excess sodium and fluid from the body. This can lead to fluid retention, which increases the volume of blood in the bloodstream and raises blood pressure.

• **Activation of the renin-angiotensin-aldosterone system (RAAS):** The kidneys produce hormones that regulate blood pressure through the RAAS. When the kidneys are damaged, this system may become overactive, causing the blood vessels to constrict and further increasing blood pressure.

This two-way relationship between CKD and hypertension makes it crucial to manage blood pressure effectively in people with kidney disease. Controlling blood pressure not only helps prevent further kidney damage but also reduces the risk of cardiovascular complications, such as heart disease and stroke.

The Importance of Early Detection and Management

One of the challenges of managing CKD is that both CKD and hypertension are often "silent" diseases in their early stages, meaning they don't always cause noticeable symptoms. This is why regular monitoring of blood pressure and kidney function is so important, especially for people at risk of CKD, such as those with diabetes or a family history of kidney disease.

- **Early intervention:** Detecting high blood pressure early allows for prompt treatment, which can slow the progression of CKD and reduce the risk of complications. Medications, lifestyle changes, and dietary adjustments can all help control blood pressure and protect the kidneys from further damage.
- **Monitoring kidney health:** For people with CKD, regular blood pressure checks, as well as tests for kidney function (such as measuring creatinine levels and glomerular filtration rate, or GFR), are essential to assess how well the kidneys are functioning and adjust treatments as needed.

The Cardiovascular Risks of Uncontrolled Blood Pressure in CKD

People with CKD are at a higher risk of cardiovascular disease, including heart attack, stroke, and heart failure. This is because uncontrolled high blood pressure can damage not only the kidneys but also the blood vessels and heart. In fact, cardiovascular disease is the leading cause of death in people with CKD.

- **Damage to blood vessels:** High blood pressure causes the arteries to become stiff and narrow, which reduces blood flow to vital organs, including the heart and brain. This can lead to heart disease, stroke, and other complications.
- **Increased workload on the heart:** When blood pressure is consistently high, the heart has to work harder to pump blood throughout the body. Over time, this can lead to thickening of the heart muscle (left ventricular hypertrophy) and eventually heart failure.

Managing blood pressure is therefore crucial not only for protecting kidney function but also for reducing the risk of serious cardiovascular events. Effective blood pressure control can significantly improve the long-term outcomes for people with CKD.

Blood Pressure Targets for People with CKD

For people with CKD, blood pressure management is typically more stringent than for the general population. The goal is to reduce the pressure on the kidneys and prevent further damage.

- **Target blood pressure:** Most guidelines recommend aiming for a blood pressure of less than 130/80 mm Hg for people with CKD, although individual targets may vary based on other health factors, such as diabetes or heart disease.
- **Regular monitoring:** Blood pressure should be monitored regularly, both at home and during doctor visits, to ensure it stays within the target range. This allows for adjustments to medications and lifestyle changes as needed.

Medications and Lifestyle Tips to Keep Your Blood Pressure in Check

For people with Chronic Kidney Disease (CKD), managing blood pressure is critical for protecting kidney function and preventing complications. A combination of medications and lifestyle changes can help keep blood pressure within a healthy range and reduce the strain on the kidneys. This section will explore the medications commonly used to control blood pressure in CKD and the lifestyle adjustments that can further support blood pressure management.

Several classes of medications are commonly prescribed to help control blood pressure in people with CKD. These medications not only lower blood pressure but also offer protective benefits for the kidneys.

ACE INHIBITORS (ANGIOTENSIN-CONVERTING ENZYME INHIBITORS)

- **How they work:** ACE inhibitors, such as lisinopril or enalapril, block the enzyme that produces angiotensin II, a hormone that narrows blood vessels. By preventing the production of angiotensin II, ACE inhibitors help blood vessels relax, lowering blood pressure and reducing the strain on the kidneys.
- **Kidney protection:** ACE inhibitors are particularly beneficial for people with CKD because they help reduce proteinuria (the leakage of protein into the urine), which is a sign of kidney damage. By lowering blood pressure and

reducing proteinuria, ACE inhibitors can slow the progression of CKD.

ARBs (Angiotensin II Receptor Blockers)

- **How they work:** ARBs, such as losartan or valsartan, block the action of angiotensin II rather than its production. By preventing angiotensin II from binding to its receptors in the blood vessels, ARBs help the vessels relax, lowering blood pressure.
- **Kidney protection:** Like ACE inhibitors, ARBs help reduce proteinuria and protect the kidneys from further damage. They are often used as an alternative to ACE inhibitors if the patient experiences side effects like a persistent cough.

Diuretics (Water Pills)

Diuretics, such as furosemide or hydrochlorothiazide, help the body eliminate excess sodium and water by increasing urine production. This reduces the volume of fluid in the bloodstream, which helps lower blood pressure.

Managing fluid retention

Diuretics are especially helpful for people with CKD who experience fluid retention (edema), as they help reduce swelling and prevent fluid overload. However, diuretics can also affect electrolyte levels, so regular monitoring is necessary.

Beta Blockers

Beta blockers, such as metoprolol or atenolol, reduce the workload on the heart by slowing the heart rate and lowering blood pressure. They are often prescribed to people with CKD who also have heart disease.

Beta blockers are typically used when blood pressure is not adequately controlled with ACE inhibitors, ARBs, or diuretics, or when heart-related complications need to be addressed.

Calcium Channel Blockers

Calcium channel blockers, such as amlodipine or diltiazem, relax the muscles in the walls of blood vessels, allowing them to widen and lower blood pressure.

How they are used in CKD

Calcium channel blockers may be added to the treatment regimen when blood pressure control requires additional support or if the patient cannot tolerate ACE inhibitors or ARBs.

Aldosterone Antagonists

Medications like spironolactone block the action of aldosterone, a hormone that causes the kidneys to retain sodium and water. By blocking aldosterone, these medications help reduce fluid retention and lower blood pressure.

Aldosterone antagonists are sometimes used in combination with other blood pressure medications, particularly in people with resistant hypertension (blood pressure that is difficult to control).

Lifestyle Tips for Managing Blood Pressure in CKD

In addition to medications, certain lifestyle changes can help support blood pressure control and improve overall kidney health. These changes are especially important for reducing the need for higher doses of medications and improving long-term outcomes.

Reduce Sodium Intake

Excess sodium causes the body to retain water, which increases blood pressure and puts extra strain on the kidneys. Reducing sodium intake can help lower blood pressure and prevent fluid retention.

How to reduce sodium

Aim for no more than 1,500-2,000 mg of sodium per day. This can be achieved by avoiding processed and packaged foods, which often contain high levels of sodium, and opting for fresh, whole foods instead. Use herbs, spices, and lemon juice to flavor food instead of salt.

Maintain a Healthy Weight

Being overweight increases the risk of high blood pressure, which can worsen kidney damage. Losing even a small amount of weight can help reduce blood pressure and improve overall health.

How to maintain a healthy weight

Focus on a balanced diet rich in fruits, vegetables, lean proteins, and whole grains. Regular physical activity, such as walking, swimming, or yoga, can also help manage weight and improve cardiovascular health.

Exercise Regularly

Regular physical activity helps lower blood pressure by improving circulation, reducing stress, and promoting overall cardiovascular health. It also helps with weight management, which can further support blood pressure control.

How to incorporate exercise

Aim for at least 150 minutes of moderate-intensity exercise per week, such as brisk walking or cycling. If you're new to exercise, start slowly and gradually increase the duration and intensity of your workouts. Always check with your healthcare provider before starting a new exercise routine, especially if you have advanced CKD.

Limit Alcohol Intake

Drinking too much alcohol can raise blood pressure and contribute to weight gain, both of which are harmful to kidney health.

If you choose to drink alcohol, do so in moderation—no more than one drink per day for women and two drinks per day for men. Avoid binge drinking, as it can cause significant spikes in blood pressure.

Quit Smoking

Smoking damages blood vessels, raises blood pressure, and increases the risk of heart disease—all of which are harmful to people with CKD.

Quitting smoking is one of the best things you can do for your overall health, including your kidneys. If you need help quitting, talk to your healthcare provider about smoking cessation programs, medications, or nicotine replacement therapy.

Manage Stress

Chronic stress can raise blood pressure and contribute to poor health outcomes in people with CKD. Finding ways to manage stress can help lower blood pressure and improve emotional well-being.

How to manage Stress

Incorporate relaxation techniques like meditation, deep breathing exercises, yoga, or Tai Chi into your routine. Spending time in nature, connecting with loved ones, and practicing mindfulness can also help reduce stress.

Monitoring Blood Pressure

Regular blood pressure monitoring is essential for people with CKD to ensure that their blood pressure remains within the target range.

- **Home monitoring:** Consider using a home blood pressure monitor to track your blood pressure between doctor visits. This allows you to identify patterns and make adjustments to your lifestyle or medications as needed.
- **Doctor visits:** Regular check-ups with your healthcare provider are important for assessing your blood pressure, kidney function, and overall health. Your doctor may adjust your medications based on your blood pressure readings and other factors.

Anemia and Fatigue

Understanding Why CKD Leads to Low Energy Levels

Chronic Kidney Disease (CKD) often leads to persistent fatigue and low energy levels, which can significantly affect a person's quality of life. Many individuals with CKD experience constant tiredness, difficulty staying alert, and a lack of motivation or physical strength. This exhaustion is not simply a result of having a chronic illness; several underlying factors contribute to the fatigue experienced by CKD patients. Understanding these causes can help in managing and treating fatigue effectively.

Anemia: A Major Cause of Fatigue in CKD

One of the primary reasons people with CKD feel fatigued is anemia, a condition in which the body does not have enough red blood cells to carry oxygen to the tissues. The kidneys play a crucial role in producing a hormone called erythropoietin (EPO), which stimulates the bone marrow to produce red blood cells. When the kidneys are damaged, they produce less EPO, leading to a reduced number of red blood cells and, consequently, anemia.

- **Why anemia causes fatigue**: Red blood cells are responsible for transporting oxygen from the lungs to the rest of the body. When there aren't enough red blood cells, less oxygen reaches the tissues and organs. This lack of oxygen makes the muscles and brain work harder, leading to feelings of fatigue, weakness, and exhaustion.

- **Symptoms of anemia:** In addition to fatigue, anemia can cause symptoms such as shortness of breath, dizziness, pale skin, and a rapid heartbeat. Many people with CKD don't realize they have anemia until these symptoms become noticeable.

Toxin Buildup Due to Reduced Kidney Function

As CKD progresses, the kidneys become less effective at filtering waste products and toxins from the blood. This leads to a buildup of urea, creatinine, and other waste products that would normally be excreted through urine. The accumulation of these toxins in the bloodstream, known as uremia, can lead to various symptoms, including fatigue.

- **Why toxin buildup causes fatigue:** When waste products accumulate in the blood, they disrupt normal cellular function, leading to inflammation, reduced energy production, and an overall feeling of malaise. The brain and muscles, in particular, are affected by the presence of toxins, which contributes to mental and physical fatigue.
- BOther symptoms of toxin buildup: In addition to fatigue, uremia can cause nausea, vomiting, difficulty concentrating (also known as "brain fog"), and an overall sense of feeling unwell. These symptoms may worsen as kidney function declines.

Fluid and Electrolyte Imbalances

People with CKD often experience fluid retention and electrolyte imbalances, which can further contribute to feelings of fatigue and exhaustion. When the kidneys are not functioning properly, they have difficulty regulating the balance of fluids and electrolytes, such as sodium, potassium, and calcium.

- Fluid retention and swelling: As kidney function declines, excess fluid may accumulate in the body, leading to swelling in the legs, ankles, and feet. This added fluid can make you feel heavier and more sluggish, contributing to feelings of fatigue.
- Electrolyte imbalances: Imbalances in electrolytes can interfere with normal muscle and nerve function, leading to muscle weakness, cramps, and lethargy. For example, too much potassium (hyperkalemia) or too little sodium (hyponatremia) can make you feel tired and drained of energy.

Inflammation and Immune Response

Chronic inflammation is a common issue in people with CKD. The body's immune system is often in a heightened state due to the presence of waste products and toxins that the kidneys are unable to filter out effectively. This persistent immune response leads to the release of inflammatory cytokines, chemicals that cause inflammation and fatigue.

- Why inflammation causes fatigue: Inflammation affects how cells produce and use energy. When inflammatory cytokines are constantly elevated, they interfere with the body's ability to produce ATP (the primary energy source for cells), leading to a reduction in overall energy levels. Inflammation also contributes to muscle and joint pain, which can further exacerbate fatigue.
- Systemic effects of inflammation: The chronic inflammation associated with CKD doesn't just affect the kidneys; it impacts the entire body. This can lead to other symptoms, such as joint pain, digestive issues, and an increased risk of cardiovascular disease, all of which can drain energy and lead to feelings of exhaustion.

Sleep Disturbances in CKD

Many people with CKD experience sleep disturbances, which can significantly impact energy levels and contribute to daytime fatigue. Several factors related to CKD can interfere with getting a restful night's sleep:

- Nocturia: Frequent urination during the night (nocturia) is common in people with CKD, particularly in the later stages. Having to wake up multiple times during the night to urinate can disrupt sleep cycles and lead to fatigue during the day.
- Restless Legs Syndrome (RLS): Restless Legs Syndrome, a condition that causes uncomfortable sensations in the legs and an irresistible urge to move them, is more common in people with CKD. RLS often occurs in the evening or at night, making it difficult to fall asleep or stay asleep.
- Sleep apnea: Sleep apnea, a condition in which breathing repeatedly stops and starts during sleep, is more prevalent in people with CKD. It leads to poor sleep quality and contributes to feelings of fatigue and lack of energy during the day.
- Insomnia: Many people with CKD experience insomnia, either due to anxiety about their condition, discomfort from fluid retention, or side effects of medications. Insomnia can make it difficult to get enough sleep, leaving individuals feeling drained and lethargic.

Nutritional Deficiencies

People with CKD often have to follow a restricted diet to limit certain nutrients that can be harmful to the kidneys, such as sodium, potassium, and phosphorus. However, this can sometimes lead to nutritional deficiencies that contribute to low energy levels.

- **Iron deficiency:** Iron is essential for producing hemoglobin, the protein in red blood cells that carries oxygen. A lack of iron can lead to anemia, further exacerbating feelings of fatigue. Many people with CKD are at risk for iron deficiency, either due to dietary restrictions or because the kidneys are less able to absorb and utilize iron effectively.

- **B-vitamin deficiencies:** B vitamins, particularly B12 and folate, are crucial for energy production and red blood cell formation. Deficiencies in these vitamins can contribute to fatigue and weakness. Some people with CKD may have difficulty absorbing or maintaining adequate levels of B vitamins.

- **Protein-energy wasting:** In advanced stages of CKD, protein-energy wasting (PEW) can occur, leading to muscle loss, weakness, and fatigue. PEW is characterized by a loss of muscle mass and fat due to poor nutrition, inflammation, and the body's inability to use protein efficiently.

Medications and Supplements to Manage Anemia

Anemia is one of the leading causes of fatigue in people with Chronic Kidney Disease (CKD). When the kidneys are damaged, they produce less erythropoietin (EPO), a hormone that stimulates the production of red blood cells. As a result, people with CKD often develop anemia, which contributes to persistent tiredness, weakness, and reduced energy levels. Managing anemia through medications and supplements is crucial for improving quality of life and slowing the progression of CKD.

1. ERYTHROPOIESIS-STIMULATING AGENTS (ESAs)

One of the most common treatments for anemia in CKD is the use of erythropoiesis-stimulating agents (ESAs). These medications mimic the action of erythropoietin, the hormone normally produced by the kidneys, to encourage the production of red blood cells in the bone marrow.

- **How ESAs work:** ESAs are synthetic forms of erythropoietin that help stimulate the bone marrow to produce more red blood cells, increasing the oxygen-carrying capacity of the blood and reducing symptoms of anemia such as fatigue and weakness.
- **Common ESAs:** Some commonly used ESAs include epoetin alfa (Epogen, Procrit) and darbepoetin alfa (Aranesp). These medications are typically administered via injection under the skin or into a vein, and your doctor will determine the appropriate dose based on your hemoglobin levels and kidney function.

- **Monitoring and risks:** While ESAs can effectively manage anemia, they must be carefully monitored to avoid complications. Overuse of ESAs can lead to excessively high hemoglobin levels, which increases the risk of stroke, heart attack, and blood clots. Regular blood tests are necessary to ensure that your hemoglobin stays within a safe range.

2. IRON SUPPLEMENTS

Iron deficiency is a common cause of anemia in people with CKD. Since iron is essential for producing hemoglobin, the protein in red blood cells that carries oxygen, low levels of iron can exacerbate anemia. Iron supplements are often prescribed to replenish iron stores and improve red blood cell production.

- **Oral iron supplements:** Ferrous sulfate, ferrous gluconate, and ferrous fumarate are commonly prescribed oral iron supplements. These are taken by mouth and help boost iron levels in the bloodstream. However, some people with CKD may have difficulty absorbing iron through the digestive system, and oral iron supplements can sometimes cause gastrointestinal side effects like constipation, nausea, or stomach upset.
- **Intravenous (IV) iron:** For individuals who cannot tolerate oral iron or do not respond well to it, intravenous (IV) iron infusions may be used. Iron sucrose (Venofer) and iron dextran (INFeD) are examples of IV iron treatments that deliver iron directly into the bloodstream, bypassing the digestive system. IV iron is often administered in a clinic or hospital setting and can more effectively raise iron levels in people with CKD.

- **Monitoring and side effects:** Iron supplements, whether oral or intravenous, require careful monitoring. Too much iron can cause toxicity and damage organs, including the liver and heart. Regular blood tests will be conducted to monitor iron levels and ensure they remain within a safe range.

3. VITAMIN B12 AND FOLATE SUPPLEMENTS

Vitamin B12 and folate (vitamin B9) are essential nutrients for the production of red blood cells. Deficiencies in these vitamins can contribute to anemia, particularly in people with CKD who may have difficulty absorbing these nutrients.

- **Vitamin B12 supplements:** Vitamin B12 is found in animal products like meat, eggs, and dairy, but some people with CKD may not get enough B12 from their diet, especially if they follow a restricted or vegetarian diet. Cyanocobalamin or methylcobalamin are commonly used forms of B12 supplements, which can be taken orally or administered via injection.
- **Folate supplements:** Folate is another important B vitamin that helps produce red blood cells. Folate deficiency can lead to megaloblastic anemia, a condition where red blood cells are abnormally large and unable to function properly. Folic acid supplements can help correct this deficiency and improve red blood cell production.
- **Importance of monitoring:** Like iron, B12 and folate levels should be monitored regularly through blood tests to ensure you're getting enough of these nutrients without taking too much.

4. **Vitamin D Supplements**

Vitamin D plays a role in regulating the production of red blood cells and maintaining bone health. In CKD, impaired kidney function leads to reduced activation of vitamin D, which can contribute to both anemia and bone-related complications.

- **Activated vitamin D:** In people with CKD, the kidneys are unable to convert vitamin D into its active form, calcitriol. For this reason, people with CKD often need supplements of activated vitamin D or vitamin D analogs, such as calcitriol, paricalcitol, or doxercalciferol. These supplements help support red blood cell production and improve overall health.
- **Vitamin D monitoring:** It's important to work with your healthcare provider to determine the right dose of vitamin D, as too much can lead to elevated calcium levels, which can cause other complications.

5. **Reducing Inflammation with Anti-Inflammatory Supplements**

Chronic inflammation, which is common in CKD, can interfere with the body's ability to produce red blood cells, contributing to anemia. Certain anti-inflammatory supplements may help reduce inflammation and improve anemia symptoms.

- **Omega-3 fatty acids:** Found in fish oil, omega-3s have anti-inflammatory properties that may help reduce inflammation and support overall health. While omega-3s do not directly treat anemia, reducing inflammation can help the body respond better to treatments like ESAs and iron supplements.

- **Turmeric:** Curcumin, the active ingredient in turmeric, has been shown to have anti-inflammatory effects. Like omega-3s, turmeric can help lower inflammation, which may indirectly improve anemia management.

Lifestyle Adjustments to Manage Anemia

In addition to medications and supplements, certain lifestyle changes can help manage anemia and improve energy levels.

- **Eating a balanced, nutrient-rich diet:** Consuming foods rich in iron, vitamin B12, and folate, such as lean meats, leafy green vegetables, eggs, and fortified cereals, can help support red blood cell production. However, people with CKD must be mindful of dietary restrictions related to potassium, phosphorus, and protein, so working with a dietitian is essential.
- **Regular physical activity:** While fatigue may make exercise difficult, regular physical activity can improve circulation, reduce inflammation, and increase energy levels. Start with light activities like walking or yoga, and gradually increase your activity level as your energy improves.
- **Staying hydrated:** Proper hydration is important for overall health and helps your body function more efficiently. However, people with CKD may need to limit their fluid intake to prevent fluid retention. Follow your healthcare provider's recommendations for managing fluid intake.

Bone and Mineral Health

How CKD Affects Your Bones and What to Do About It

Chronic Kidney Disease (CKD) doesn't just affect the kidneys—it can also have a significant impact on bone health. As kidney function declines, the body's ability to regulate essential minerals like calcium and phosphorus becomes impaired, which can lead to weakened bones, an increased risk of fractures, and a condition known as Chronic Kidney Disease-Mineral and Bone Disorder (CKD-MBD). This section will explain how CKD affects your bones and what you can do to protect your bone health as part of managing your condition.

1. **Understanding Chronic Kidney Disease-Mineral and Bone Disorder (CKD-MBD)**

CKD-MBD is a common complication of chronic kidney disease that affects the bones, blood vessels, and the balance of minerals in the body. It occurs when the kidneys lose the ability to maintain proper levels of calcium, phosphorus, and vitamin D, which are crucial for bone health. This leads to abnormal bone turnover, weak bones, and an increased risk of cardiovascular problems due to calcium and phosphorus buildup in blood vessels.

- **Mineral imbalances:** Healthy kidneys help balance calcium and phosphorus levels by filtering excess phosphorus from the blood and activating vitamin D, which helps the body absorb calcium. In CKD, the kidneys cannot effectively filter phosphorus, leading to high levels of phosphorus in the blood (hyperphosphatemia). At the same time, reduced vitamin D activation leads to low calcium levels (hypocalcemia), which causes the parathyroid glands to release more parathyroid hormone (PTH) to compensate. Over time, this cycle results in weakened bones and a condition called secondary hyperparathyroidism.

- **Bone disease:** CKD-MBD can result in various types of bone disease, including:

Osteitis fibrosa cystica: A condition caused by secondary hyperparathyroidism, where high PTH levels lead to increased bone turnover, bone loss, and the formation of cyst-like areas in the bones.

Adynamic bone disease: A condition in which bones do not undergo normal turnover or repair, leading to weak and brittle bones.

Osteomalacia: A softening of the bones due to insufficient calcium and vitamin D, which can cause bone pain and increase the risk of fractures.

How CKD Affects Calcium, Phosphorus, and Vitamin D

Maintaining a proper balance of calcium, phosphorus, and vitamin D is essential for healthy bones. When kidney function declines, these nutrients become imbalanced, leading to bone and mineral disorders.

Phosphorus and Bone Health

Phosphorus is a mineral that plays an important role in forming and maintaining healthy bones and teeth. However, when phosphorus levels become too high, it can combine with calcium to form deposits in soft tissues and blood vessels, leading to vascular calcification and increasing the risk of heart disease.

High phosphorus in CKD

As the kidneys lose their ability to filter excess phosphorus from the blood, phosphorus levels rise. This stimulates the release of PTH, which pulls calcium from the bones to balance the phosphorus levels, leading to bone loss over time.

Calcium and Bone Health

Calcium is essential for building and maintaining strong bones and teeth, as well as for muscle function, nerve transmission, and blood clotting. Low calcium levels can lead to weakened bones and increased PTH production, further damaging bone structure.

Low calcium in CKD

CKD impairs the kidneys' ability to activate vitamin D, which is necessary for absorbing calcium from the diet. As a result, calcium levels drop, leading to increased PTH levels and the release of calcium from the bones. This process weakens the bones and contributes to CKD-MBD.

Vitamin D and Bone Health

Vitamin D is critical for calcium absorption and bone health. The kidneys are responsible for converting vitamin D into its active form, calcitriol, which helps the body absorb calcium and maintain healthy bones.

Low vitamin D in CKD

As kidney function declines, the kidneys are unable to activate sufficient amounts of vitamin D, leading to low calcium levels and the release of PTH. Without enough vitamin D, the body cannot absorb enough calcium to keep bones strong.

Symptoms of CKD-MBD and Bone Disease

In the early stages of CKD-MBD, many people may not notice symptoms. However, as the condition progresses, symptoms related to bone disease and mineral imbalances can develop, including:

- **Bone pain:** Pain in the bones or joints is a common symptom of bone disease in CKD. The pain may be dull and persistent, affecting daily activities.
- **Muscle weakness:** Low calcium levels and vitamin D deficiency can cause muscle weakness, making it difficult to move or perform physical tasks.
- **Fractures:** People with CKD-MBD are at a higher risk of fractures due to weakened bones. Even minor falls or injuries can lead to broken bones.
- **Itching:** High phosphorus levels can cause pruritus, a persistent itch that affects the skin, which is common in people with CKD-MBD.
- **Abnormal bone growth:** In severe cases of CKD-MBD, bones may develop abnormally, leading to deformities, particularly in children.

Managing Bone and Mineral Health in CKD

Managing CKD-MBD and protecting bone health requires a combination of medications, dietary changes, and lifestyle adjustments. Working closely with your healthcare provider to monitor and manage mineral levels is crucial for preventing further bone damage and maintaining overall health.

Phosphate Binders

Phosphate binders are medications that help control phosphorus levels by preventing the absorption of phosphorus from food in the digestive tract.

- **How they work:** Phosphate binders, such as calcium acetate, sevelamer, or lanthanum carbonate, bind to phosphorus in the gut, allowing it to be excreted in the stool rather than absorbed into the bloodstream. This helps lower phosphorus levels and reduces the risk of bone disease.
- **When to take them:** Phosphate binders are usually taken with meals to prevent phosphorus absorption from food.

Activated Vitamin D (Calcitriol) and Vitamin D Analogs

People with CKD often need supplements of activated vitamin D or vitamin D analogs to support calcium absorption and maintain bone health.

- **Activated vitamin D:** Medications like calcitriol (Rocaltrol) or vitamin D analogs such as paricalcitol and doxercalciferol are used to help the body absorb calcium and reduce PTH levels. These medications are essential for managing CKD-MBD.

- **Monitoring vitamin D levels:** Regular blood tests are necessary to monitor vitamin D levels and ensure the appropriate dosage of vitamin D supplements.

CALCIMIMETICS

Calcimimetics are medications that help control parathyroid hormone (PTH) levels in people with secondary hyperparathyroidism due to CKD.

- **How they work:** Cinacalcet (Sensipar) is a common calcimimetic that mimics the action of calcium, tricking the parathyroid glands into reducing PTH production. Lowering PTH levels can help protect the bones from further damage.

Dietary Changes

Adjusting your diet is an important part of managing bone and mineral health in CKD.

- **Limit phosphorus intake:** Reducing phosphorus in your diet can help control phosphorus levels and prevent further bone damage. Foods high in phosphorus, such as dairy products, red meat, processed foods, and sodas, should be limited.
- **Increase calcium intake (with caution):** While it's important to get enough calcium to support bone health, too much calcium can lead to deposits in the blood vessels and soft tissues. Calcium supplements should only be taken under the guidance of your healthcare provider, and dietary calcium should come from safe sources like leafy green vegetables or fortified non-dairy alternatives.
- **Monitor protein intake:** Protein is an essential nutrient, but excessive protein intake can increase phosphorus levels. Work with a dietitian to find the right balance of protein for your stage of CKD.

Regular Monitoring

It's important to have regular checkups with your healthcare provider to monitor your calcium, phosphorus, and PTH levels, as well as your overall bone health.

- **Blood tests:** Routine blood tests will help assess your mineral levels and guide adjustments to your treatment plan. These tests may include calcium, phosphorus, PTH, and vitamin D levels.
- **Bone density scans:** In some cases, your doctor may recommend a bone density scan (DEXA scan) to assess bone strength and determine your risk of fractures.

Calcium, Phosphorus, and Vitamin D: Balancing These Nutrients

In people with Chronic Kidney Disease (CKD), maintaining a balance of essential minerals like calcium, phosphorus, and vitamin D becomes increasingly difficult as kidney function declines. These nutrients play a critical role in bone health, and imbalances can lead to weakened bones, cardiovascular complications, and other health issues. This section will explore why balancing calcium, phosphorus, and vitamin D is crucial for people with CKD, and what can be done to manage these nutrients effectively.

Why Balancing Calcium, Phosphorus, and Vitamin D is Important

The kidneys are responsible for maintaining the balance of calcium and phosphorus in the body, as well as activating vitamin D, which helps the body absorb calcium from food. When kidney function declines, these processes are disrupted, leading to mineral imbalances that affect bone health and increase the risk of complications like Chronic Kidney Disease-Mineral and Bone Disorder (CKD-MBD).

- **Calcium:** Calcium is essential for building and maintaining strong bones and teeth, as well as for proper muscle function and nerve transmission. In CKD, calcium levels can become low due to reduced vitamin D activation, leading to bone weakness and increased risk of fractures. At the same time, the body may try to compensate by releasing calcium from the bones, which weakens them further.

- **Phosphorus:** Phosphorus is another mineral that plays a role in bone health. It works alongside calcium to form strong bones and teeth. However, in CKD, the kidneys are unable to effectively remove excess phosphorus from the blood, leading to high phosphorus levels (hyperphosphatemia). This causes calcium to be pulled from the bones, making them weak and brittle. Excess phosphorus can also bind with calcium in the bloodstream, forming deposits in soft tissues and blood vessels, which increases the risk of cardiovascular disease.

- . **Vitamin D:** Vitamin D helps regulate calcium and phosphorus levels in the blood by promoting the absorption of calcium from the intestines. In CKD, the kidneys are unable to activate vitamin D into its usable form, calcitriol, leading to low calcium levels and the stimulation of parathyroid hormone (PTH) production. High PTH levels can cause further bone loss and mineral imbalances.

Managing Phosphorus Levels

Controlling phosphorus levels is one of the most important aspects of managing mineral balance in CKD. Elevated phosphorus levels can cause serious complications, including bone disease and calcification of blood vessels and soft tissues.

Dietary Changes to Limit Phosphorus Intake

- **Limit high-phosphorus foods:** Foods that are high in phosphorus, such as dairy products, red meats, processed foods, nuts, seeds, and sodas, should be limited in people with CKD. Avoiding foods with added phosphorus (often found in processed foods and colas) is particularly important because these phosphorus additives are absorbed more easily by the body.
- **Read food labels:** Phosphorus additives are often found in processed foods and beverages, including sodas, fast foods, and some baked goods. Look for ingredients like "phosphoric acid" or "phosphate" on food labels, and try to avoid products with these additives.
- **Work with a dietitian:** A registered dietitian who specializes in CKD can help you create a kidney-friendly diet plan that limits phosphorus while ensuring you get enough nutrients to support overall health.

Phosphate Binders

For people with CKD, dietary changes alone may not be enough to control phosphorus levels. Phosphate binders are medications that help prevent the absorption of phosphorus from food in the digestive tract.

- **How phosphate binders work:** These medications bind to phosphorus in the food you eat, allowing it to be excreted in the stool rather than absorbed into the bloodstream. This helps reduce phosphorus levels in the blood and prevents further bone damage.

- **Types of phosphate binders:** There are several types of phosphate binders, including:

Calcium-based binders: These include calcium acetate and calcium carbonate, which bind to phosphorus in the gut and help lower phosphorus levels. However, calcium-based binders must be used carefully to avoid raising blood calcium levels too high.

Non-calcium-based binders: These include sevelamer (Renvela) and lanthanum carbonate (Fosrenol), which do not increase calcium levels and are often preferred for people who need to avoid excess calcium.

- **When to take phosphate binders:** Phosphate binders are usually taken with meals to prevent phosphorus from being absorbed. It's important to follow your doctor's instructions on when and how to take these medications for optimal effectiveness.

Managing Calcium Levels

Maintaining a proper balance of calcium is crucial for bone health and preventing complications in CKD. Too little calcium can lead to weak bones, while too much calcium can cause calcification of blood vessels and soft tissues.

Calcium Supplements

In some cases, people with CKD may need to take calcium supplements to maintain healthy calcium levels. However, calcium supplementation should be done under medical supervision, as too much calcium can be harmful.

- **When calcium supplements are needed:** If your blood calcium levels are too low, your doctor may recommend calcium supplements to support bone health. However, if you are also taking a calcium-based phosphate binder, your calcium intake must be carefully monitored to avoid excess calcium in the blood.
- **Avoid excessive calcium intake:** Taking too much calcium, especially through supplements, can lead to a condition called hypercalcemia (high blood calcium levels). This can cause calcium deposits to form in blood vessels, increasing the risk of heart disease and stroke. Work closely with your healthcare provider to ensure your calcium intake is appropriate for your condition.

Dietary Sources of Calcium

For people with CKD, it's important to get enough calcium to support bone health, but without overloading the body with too much.

- **Safe sources of calcium:** Low-potassium vegetables, such as kale, collard greens, and broccoli, can provide calcium without contributing to excessive phosphorus or potassium levels. Some non-dairy alternatives, like fortified almond or rice milk, are also good sources of calcium.
- **Limit high-calcium foods:** While it's important to get enough calcium, you may need to limit foods that are very high in calcium but also high in phosphorus, such as dairy products.

Managing Vitamin D Levels

Vitamin D is essential for helping the body absorb calcium and maintain bone strength. However, in CKD, the kidneys lose the ability to convert vitamin D into its active form, calcitriol, which is necessary for calcium absorption.

Activated Vitamin D Supplements
People with CKD often require activated vitamin D or vitamin D analogs to support bone health and prevent mineral imbalances.

- **Calcitriol and vitamin D analogs:** Activated vitamin D, such as calcitriol (Rocaltrol), or vitamin D analogs like paricalcitol or doxercalciferol, are used to increase calcium absorption from the gut and lower PTH levels. These medications help maintain a proper balance of calcium and phosphorus while protecting bone health.
- **Monitoring vitamin D levels:** Regular blood tests are needed to monitor vitamin D levels and adjust the dosage of supplements as necessary. Too much activated vitamin D can cause high calcium levels, so it's important to follow your doctor's instructions.

Dietary Sources of Vitamin D
While vitamin D is naturally produced by the body in response to sunlight, dietary sources can also help maintain adequate levels.

- **Foods rich in vitamin D:** Fatty fish (such as salmon and mackerel), fortified cereals, and egg yolks are good sources of vitamin D. However, it can be challenging to get enough vitamin D from food alone, especially in people with CKD, so supplements may be necessary.

Parathyroid Hormone (PTH) and Bone Health

In CKD, the imbalance of calcium, phosphorus, and vitamin D can lead to elevated levels of parathyroid hormone (PTH), a condition known as secondary hyperparathyroidism. High PTH levels cause the bones to release calcium, leading to bone loss and increasing the risk of fractures.

Calcimimetics

For people with secondary hyperparathyroidism, calcimimetics are medications that help lower PTH levels by mimicking the action of calcium in the blood.

- **How calcimimetics work:** Cinacalcet (Sensipar) is a common calcimimetic that signals the parathyroid glands to reduce PTH production. By lowering PTH levels, calcimimetics help protect bones from further damage.
- **Monitoring PTH levels:** Regular blood tests are needed to monitor PTH levels and adjust treatment as necessary. Keeping PTH within the target range can help reduce bone loss and improve overall bone health.

Managing Fluid Retention

Tips for Reducing Swelling and Controlling Fluid Intake

For people with Chronic Kidney Disease (CKD), managing fluid intake is crucial for controlling fluid retention and reducing swelling (also known as edema). As kidney function declines, the body struggles to maintain a proper balance of fluids, leading to a buildup of excess water in tissues. This can cause swelling in the legs, ankles, feet, hands, and sometimes even the face. Fluid overload can also increase blood pressure, cause difficulty breathing, and lead to other complications such as heart failure. Managing fluid intake, along with following medical advice, can help reduce these symptoms and improve overall well-being.

Here are some practical tips for reducing swelling and controlling fluid intake.

1. Limit Your Daily Fluid Intake

When the kidneys are no longer able to regulate fluid balance, it's important to limit how much fluid you consume each day to avoid fluid overload. Your doctor or dietitian will recommend a specific amount of fluid based on the stage of your CKD, your overall health, and your treatment plan (such as dialysis).

- **Work with your healthcare provider:** Your doctor or dietitian will determine how much fluid is safe for you to consume each day. This will take into account how much urine your body is still producing and whether you are on dialysis. People on dialysis may have stricter fluid limits.
- **Include all fluids:** When tracking fluid intake, remember to count not only beverages but also foods that contain a lot of water. This includes soups, broths, gelatin, popsicles, and even foods like watermelon, cucumber, and yogurt.
- **Use a fluid diary:** Keeping a daily log of your fluid intake can help you stay on track. Measure out your fluids ahead of time so you can be aware of how much you're consuming throughout the day.
- **Use Portion Control for Fluids**

If you are on a fluid restriction, it can be challenging to manage your thirst and stick to the recommended fluid limit. Portion control and spreading out your fluids throughout the day can help make it easier.

- **Sip fluids throughout the day**: Instead of drinking large amounts of fluid at one time, try sipping small amounts of water or beverages throughout the day. This can help you feel more comfortable and keep your thirst in check.
- **Use small cups or glasses**: Drinking from smaller cups can help you avoid consuming too much fluid at once. This visual trick can help you stay within your fluid allowance while still feeling like you've had enough to drink.
- **Track how much you drink**: Use a measuring cup to portion out your fluids in the morning, and keep track of what you drink throughout the day. This helps ensure you stay within your recommended fluid limit.

2. Avoid High-Sodium Foods

Sodium (salt) plays a major role in fluid retention. Eating too much sodium causes your body to hold onto more water, which leads to swelling and increases blood pressure. Reducing your sodium intake can help control fluid retention and make it easier to manage swelling.

- **Limit processed and packaged foods:** Many processed foods, such as canned soups, deli meats, frozen meals, and fast foods, contain high levels of sodium. Whenever possible, choose fresh, whole foods over packaged items.
- **Read food labels:** Look for sodium content on food labels, and aim for products labeled as "low sodium" (less than 140 mg per serving). Try to keep your total daily sodium intake below 1,500-2,000 mg, or as recommended by your doctor.
- **Flavor foods with herbs and spices**: Instead of adding salt to your meals, use herbs, spices, lemon juice, or vinegar to enhance the flavor of your food without adding sodium.

3. Monitor Your Weight Regularly

Daily weight monitoring can help you track changes in fluid retention. Rapid weight gain is often a sign of fluid overload, especially if it's accompanied by swelling in the legs, feet, or hands.

- **Weigh yourself daily:** Weigh yourself at the same time each day, preferably in the morning after using the bathroom and before eating breakfast. Keep a log of your weight to spot any trends or sudden increases.
- **Look for signs of fluid retention:** In addition to weight gain, other signs of fluid retention include swelling in the

extremities, shortness of breath, or a feeling of tightness in your skin. If you notice significant weight gain or swelling, contact your healthcare provider.

4. Stay Cool and Moisturize Your Mouth

Feeling thirsty can be one of the hardest parts of limiting fluid intake, especially if you're used to drinking more. There are several ways to reduce the sensation of thirst without consuming too much fluid.

- **Keep your mouth moist:** Sucking on ice chips, hard candies, or frozen fruit like grapes can help keep your mouth moist without adding too much liquid to your daily intake. Chewing sugar-free gum can also stimulate saliva production and reduce dry mouth.
- **Stay cool:** Heat and sweating can increase thirst, so try to stay cool in warm weather. Wear light clothing, stay in air-conditioned environments, and avoid overly warm or stuffy rooms.
- **Rinse your mouth:** Swishing water around in your mouth without swallowing can provide temporary relief from thirst. Just be careful not to swallow too much water during this process.

5. Elevate Your Legs to Reduce Swelling

If you experience swelling in your legs, ankles, or feet, elevating your legs can help reduce the buildup of fluid in these areas. This is especially important after long periods of sitting or standing.

- **Elevate your legs:** When resting or sitting, prop your legs up on a pillow or cushion so that they are elevated above the level of your heart. This helps improve circulation and reduce swelling in the lower extremities.

- **Wear compression stockings:** Compression stockings can help prevent fluid from accumulating in your legs and feet. These specially designed socks provide gentle pressure to improve circulation and reduce swelling.

6. Choose Lower-Sodium Snacks

For many people, salty snacks can increase thirst, making it harder to manage fluid intake. Opt for lower-sodium snacks that won't make you as thirsty.

- **Choose fresh fruits and vegetables:** Raw fruits and vegetables are great snack options that are low in sodium and won't make you thirsty. Just be mindful of portion sizes for high-water-content fruits and vegetables if you're on a strict fluid limit.
- **Snack on protein-rich foods:** Small portions of unsalted nuts, cheese (if permitted by your diet), or hard-boiled eggs can provide protein and satisfy hunger without adding excessive sodium.

7. Avoid Carbonated Beverages and Caffeinated Drinks

Carbonated and caffeinated drinks can make you feel more bloated or thirsty. Avoiding these types of beverages can help control your fluid intake and reduce feelings of thirst.

- **Limit soda and sparkling water:** The bubbles in carbonated drinks can increase bloating, which may contribute to discomfort if you're already retaining fluids. Opt for flat beverages instead, such as herbal teas or water (within your fluid limit).

- **Cut back on caffeine:** Caffeine can act as a diuretic, increasing urine production and leading to dehydration. This may make you feel more thirsty, which can be difficult to manage if you're on a fluid restriction. Try to limit caffeinated drinks like coffee, tea, and soda.

8. Manage Thirst with Non-Liquid Options

It's common to feel thirsty when fluid intake is restricted, but there are several non-liquid strategies you can use to help manage your thirst without consuming more fluids.

- **Chew sugar-free gum or hard candy:** Chewing sugar-free gum or sucking on sugar-free hard candies can stimulate saliva production, keeping your mouth moist and reducing the sensation of thirst.
- **Suck on ice chips or frozen fruit:** Sucking on ice chips or small pieces of frozen fruit like grapes can help keep your mouth moist without consuming too much liquid.
- **Rinse your mouth:** Swishing water around in your mouth and then spitting it out can provide temporary relief from thirst without adding to your fluid intake.

9. Monitor Fluid Retention and Symptoms

It's important to regularly monitor yourself for signs of fluid retention, especially if you have CKD. Recognizing the early signs of fluid overload can help prevent complications.

- **Check for swelling:** Swelling in the ankles, feet, legs, hands, or face is a common sign of fluid retention. If you notice any new or worsening swelling, contact your healthcare provider.
- **Monitor weight:** Sudden weight gain is often a sign of fluid buildup. Weigh yourself daily, preferably in the morning

before eating or drinking, and keep track of any significant changes. An increase in weight of more than 2-3 pounds in a day or 5 pounds in a week should be reported to your doctor.

- **Watch for shortness of breath:** If fluid retention leads to shortness of breath or difficulty breathing, seek medical attention immediately. This could indicate fluid buildup in the lungs or heart, which requires prompt treatment.

10. Work with Your Healthcare Provider

Managing fluid intake and reducing swelling requires a team effort. Your doctor or dietitian can provide personalized advice based on your specific condition, medications, and treatment plan.

- **Discuss medications:** If you're experiencing significant fluid retention, your doctor may prescribe diuretics (water pills) to help your body eliminate excess fluid. However, these medications need to be used carefully, especially in people with CKD, to avoid dehydration and electrolyte imbalances.
- **Adjust your diet:** Working with a dietitian who specializes in CKD can help you manage fluid and sodium intake while still maintaining a healthy and balanced diet.

CHAPTER EIGHT

SURGICAL AND MEDICAL PROCEDURES

Dialysis: What It Is and When It's Needed

Types of Dialysis: Hemodialysis vs. Peritoneal Dialysis
When kidney function declines to a point where dialysis becomes necessary, patients and their healthcare teams must decide which type of dialysis is most suitable for their lifestyle, health status, and preferences. The two main types of dialysis are hemodialysis and peritoneal dialysis, and each has its own set of benefits, risks, and practical considerations. Understanding the differences between these two types of dialysis is important for making an informed decision about your care.

1. Hemodialysis
Hemodialysis is the most common form of dialysis. In this method, a machine filters the patient's blood outside the body, cleanses it of waste products, and then returns the purified blood back to the body. The procedure usually takes place in a

clinical setting, but in some cases, patients may undergo hemodialysis at home.

How Hemodialysis Works

- **Vascular access:** For hemodialysis to work, a reliable way to access your bloodstream is required. This is usually done through a fistula, graft, or catheter:

Arteriovenous (AV) fistula: A surgeon connects an artery to a vein, usually in the arm, creating a strong blood vessel that can handle repeated needle insertions.

Graft: If the veins aren't strong enough for a fistula, a plastic tube called a graft may be used to connect an artery to a vein.

Central venous catheter: For short-term use, a catheter may be placed in a large vein, typically in the neck or chest, though this is generally not preferred for long-term treatment.

- **Dialyzer (artificial kidney):** During hemodialysis, your blood is passed through a dialyzer, where it is filtered through a semipermeable membrane. The dialyzer removes waste, extra chemicals, and fluids from your blood, which are then disposed of.

- **Frequency and duration:** Hemodialysis typically takes 3 to 5 hours per session and is usually performed three times a week. The treatment is commonly done in a dialysis clinic or hospital, but home hemodialysis is an option for some patients, which may allow for more flexibility.

Pros and Cons of Hemodialysis
Pros:
- **Clinically supervised:** Hemodialysis performed in a clinic is managed by trained healthcare professionals, which ensures immediate assistance if complications arise.

- **Less frequent daily management:** Because treatments are typically done three times a week, patients have days off from dialysis and fewer daily responsibilities related to treatment.

Cons:

- **Time-consuming:** Each session takes several hours, and patients must travel to a dialysis center multiple times a week.
- **Possible discomfort:** Insertion of needles into the fistula or graft can be uncomfortable, and some patients experience cramping or blood pressure changes during treatment.
- **Inflexible schedule:** For those undergoing dialysis at a clinic, the treatment schedule can be rigid, which may interfere with work, travel, or personal activities.

2. Peritoneal Dialysis

Peritoneal dialysis (PD) uses the lining of your abdomen (the peritoneal membrane) as a filter to remove waste and excess fluid from your body. This method allows for more independence and flexibility, as it can often be done at home and during daily activities.

How Peritoneal Dialysis Works
- **Catheter placement:** A soft tube called a peritoneal dialysis catheter is surgically placed into the patient's abdomen. This catheter provides access to the peritoneal cavity, where the dialysis solution (dialysate) is infused.
- **Dialysis process:** A sterile solution called dialysate is infused into the peritoneal cavity through the catheter. The solution absorbs waste products and excess fluids from the blood vessels in the peritoneal lining. After a few hours, the solution is drained from the body and replaced with fresh dialysate. This process is called an exchange.

Two methods of peritoneal dialysis:

Continuous Ambulatory Peritoneal Dialysis (CAPD): This method involves manual exchanges of dialysate several times a day, typically every 4 to 6 hours. Each exchange takes about 30-40 minutes, and the patient can continue normal activities between exchanges.

Automated Peritoneal Dialysis (APD): This method uses a machine called a cycler to perform exchanges automatically, usually overnight while the patient sleeps. APD allows for greater flexibility during the day.

Pros and Cons of Peritoneal Dialysis

Pros:
- **Flexibility and independence:** Peritoneal dialysis can be done at home, allowing patients to maintain their daily routines and independence. APD, in particular, frees up daytime hours.
- **Gentler on the body:** Because peritoneal dialysis is continuous, fluid and waste are removed more gradually than with hemodialysis, which can be easier on the heart and body.
- **No needles:** Unlike hemodialysis, peritoneal dialysis does not require needles, which may be more comfortable for some patients.

Cons:
- **Infection risk:** There is a risk of infection at the catheter site or in the peritoneal cavity (peritonitis). Patients must be diligent about hygiene and proper technique to avoid infections.
- **. Daily responsibility:** Peritoneal dialysis requires daily management, and patients or caregivers must be trained to perform exchanges or operate the cycler.
- **Less effective for some patients:** In certain cases, peritoneal dialysis may not be as effective at removing fluid and waste as hemodialysis, particularly for patients with larger body sizes or severe kidney failure.

Choosing Between Hemodialysis and Peritoneal Dialysis

The choice between hemodialysis and peritoneal dialysis depends on a variety of factors, including the patient's lifestyle, medical condition, personal preferences, and support system.

- **Lifestyle considerations:** Patients who prefer more flexibility and independence may opt for peritoneal dialysis, while those who prefer clinical supervision and fewer daily responsibilities may choose hemodialysis.
- **Medical factors:** Some medical conditions, such as abdominal surgeries or infections, may make peritoneal dialysis less suitable. Similarly, patients with certain cardiovascular conditions may benefit from the slower, gentler fluid removal of peritoneal dialysis.
- **Support system:** Home dialysis, whether hemodialysis or peritoneal, requires a supportive environment and proper training. Patients need to feel comfortable managing their treatment or have a caregiver who can assist.

What to Expect if Dialysis Becomes Necessary

When dialysis becomes necessary, it's important to understand what the treatment involves and how it will impact your day-to-day life. Whether you undergo hemodialysis or peritoneal dialysis, the process can seem overwhelming at first, but with the right support and preparation, it can become a manageable part of your routine. This section will walk you through what to expect when starting dialysis, including how to prepare, what the treatments are like, and how to adapt to life on dialysis.

Preparing for Dialysis

Before starting dialysis, your healthcare team will take several steps to prepare your body and ensure that you are ready for treatment. The type of preparation will depend on whether you're starting hemodialysis or peritoneal dialysis.

For Hemodialysis: Vascular Access Preparation

One of the first steps in preparing for hemodialysis is creating a vascular access point, which is where your blood will be drawn from and returned to during treatment. This is typically done through surgery, and the type of access you receive will depend on your overall health and the condition of your veins.

- **Arteriovenous (AV) Fistula:** An AV fistula is the preferred type of access for most people because it's the most durable and has the lowest risk of infection. A surgeon will connect an artery to a vein, usually in your arm, to create a strong blood vessel that can handle repeated needle insertions for dialysis.

- **Arteriovenous (AV) Graft:** If your veins are too small or weak for a fistula, a graft may be used instead. This is a synthetic tube that connects an artery to a vein, allowing for blood flow during dialysis.
- **Central Venous Catheter:** In emergency situations or when dialysis is needed quickly, a catheter may be placed in a large vein, usually in your neck or chest. This is typically a temporary solution, as long-term catheters have a higher risk of infection and other complications.

For Peritoneal Dialysis: Catheter Placement

If you are opting for peritoneal dialysis, a catheter will need to be placed in your abdomen. This is a soft, flexible tube that will allow the dialysate solution to flow in and out of your peritoneal cavity during treatment.

- **Surgical procedure:** The catheter is placed during a minor surgical procedure, usually done under local or general anesthesia. It will take a few weeks for the catheter site to heal before you can start peritoneal dialysis, so early planning is important.
- **Training for home dialysis:** Once your catheter is placed and you're ready to start treatment, you'll receive training on how to perform peritoneal dialysis at home. You'll learn how to maintain a sterile environment, perform exchanges, and monitor for signs of infection.

What Happens During Dialysis

Each dialysis session is designed to mimic the function of healthy kidneys by filtering waste products, excess fluids, and toxins from the blood. Here's what to expect during the treatment process for both hemodialysis and peritoneal dialysis.

Hemodialysis

If you're receiving hemodialysis at a clinic, you'll arrive for your scheduled session, which typically occurs three times a week. Each session lasts about 3 to 5 hours, so it's important to plan accordingly.

Once you're seated, the nurse or technician will connect you to the dialysis machine by inserting two needles into your vascular access (fistula or graft). One needle will remove your blood to be filtered, and the other will return the cleaned blood to your body. If you have a catheter, the blood will flow through the catheter without the need for needles.

As your blood flows through the dialysis machine, waste products, excess fluids, and toxins are removed by the dialyzer. During the treatment, you can relax, read, watch TV, or rest. Some patients experience mild discomfort, such as muscle cramps or changes in blood pressure, but these can usually be managed by the clinic staff.

After the dialysis session is complete, the needles will be removed, and you'll be monitored for a short time before heading home. You may feel tired afterward, but this usually improves as your body adjusts to the treatment over time.

Peritoneal Dialysis

Peritoneal dialysis can be done at home, either manually (Continuous Ambulatory Peritoneal Dialysis, or CAPD) or using a machine (Automated Peritoneal Dialysis, or APD). You'll learn how to perform exchanges, which involve draining old dialysate from your abdomen and replacing it with fresh dialysate. CAPD exchanges are done several times a day, while APD is typically done overnight while you sleep.

It's important to keep the area around the catheter clean and dry to prevent infection. You'll be trained on how to care for the catheter site and monitor for signs of infection, such as redness, swelling, or fever.

Peritoneal dialysis offers more flexibility than hemodialysis because it can be done at home and doesn't require frequent trips to a clinic. However, it requires daily management and a strict adherence to your dialysis schedule.

Managing Side Effects

Dialysis can cause some side effects, though they vary depending on the type of dialysis and the individual. It's important to be aware of these potential issues and work with your healthcare team to manage them.

- **Fatigue:** Many people feel tired after dialysis sessions, particularly in the early stages of treatment. This often improves as your body adjusts, but it's important to rest when needed and maintain a healthy diet to support your energy levels.
- **Low blood pressure:** Sudden drops in blood pressure can occur during hemodialysis, leading to dizziness, nausea, or fainting. Staying hydrated between sessions and following

your doctor's advice on diet and fluid intake can help manage this.

- **Muscle cramps:** Muscle cramps are a common side effect of hemodialysis, usually due to fluid removal. Adjusting your dialysis prescription or fluid intake can often reduce the frequency of cramps.
- **Infection risks:** Peritoneal dialysis carries a risk of infection, particularly peritonitis (infection of the abdominal lining). It's essential to follow proper hygiene protocols and seek immediate medical attention if you notice signs of infection.

4. Adjusting to Life on Dialysis

Dialysis is a significant adjustment, both physically and emotionally. However, with time and support, many people are able to adapt and continue leading fulfilling lives. Here are some tips for adjusting to life on dialysis:

- **Stay informed:** Understanding your treatment and being involved in your care can help you feel more in control. Ask your healthcare team questions, attend educational sessions, and keep up with the latest information about dialysis and kidney disease.
- **Maintain a healthy diet:** Following a kidney-friendly diet is essential to managing your condition and feeling your best. Your dietitian will help you adjust your diet to control fluid intake, manage electrolytes, and maintain proper nutrition.
- **Stay active:** While dialysis may make you feel fatigued at first, staying physically active can help improve your energy levels, strengthen your muscles, and enhance your overall well-being. Start with light activities like walking or yoga and build up your endurance over time.

- **Seek emotional support:** Adjusting to life on dialysis can be emotionally challenging. It's important to talk about your feelings with loved ones, join a support group, or consider counseling to help you cope with the changes in your life.

Regular Monitoring and Adjustments

Throughout your time on dialysis, your healthcare team will regularly monitor your health, lab results, and treatment plan to ensure your dialysis is effective and that you're staying as healthy as possible.

- **Blood tests:** Regular blood tests will be performed to monitor your potassium, phosphorus, calcium, and other important levels. Your dialysis prescription may be adjusted based on these results.
- **Ongoing care:** You'll continue to work closely with your nephrologist, dietitian, and dialysis team to make sure your treatment is optimized and any side effects or complications are managed.

Kidney Transplant: A Long-Term Solution

Understanding How Kidney Transplant Works

A kidney transplant is often considered the best long-term treatment option for people with end-stage renal disease (ESRD) or advanced Chronic Kidney Disease (CKD), as it offers a chance for improved quality of life and independence from dialysis. A kidney transplant involves replacing a person's failed kidneys with a healthy kidney from a living or deceased donor. For many patients, a successful kidney transplant can lead to a longer and healthier life, with greater freedom in daily activities and fewer dietary and fluid restrictions compared to dialysis.

This section will explore how kidney transplants work, the surgical process, and the considerations involved in this life-changing procedure.

How Does a Kidney Transplant Work?

A kidney transplant involves surgically placing a healthy kidney from a donor into the recipient's body to take over the functions that the failed kidneys can no longer perform. The new kidney will filter blood, remove waste, and balance fluids and electrolytes, just as healthy kidneys would.

- **Donor kidney:** The donor kidney can come from a living donor (such as a relative or friend) or a deceased donor. Living donor transplants tend to have better outcomes and shorter waiting times, but both types of donations can be successful.

- **Recipient's kidneys:** In most cases, the recipient's diseased kidneys are not removed during the transplant. The new kidney is placed in the lower abdomen, near the pelvis, and connected to the recipient's blood vessels and bladder. The new kidney will begin to function soon after the transplant, allowing the body to eliminate waste and maintain fluid balance.

Who is Eligible for a Transplant and How to Get on the List

A kidney transplant can provide a better quality of life and long-term survival for many people with end-stage renal disease (ESRD). However, not everyone is eligible for a kidney transplant, and the process of getting on the transplant list can be complex. Eligibility for a transplant depends on several medical and non-medical factors, including your overall health, the stage of your kidney disease, and your ability to adhere to the post-transplant care required to keep the new kidney functioning.

This section will explain who is eligible for a kidney transplant, the process of getting on the transplant list, and alternative options if a living donor is available.

To be eligible for a kidney transplant, you must meet certain medical criteria that ensure your body is healthy enough to undergo surgery and manage the necessary post-transplant care. Your eligibility will be determined by a transplant evaluation, which involves a series of medical tests, consultations, and discussions with your healthcare team.

Eligibility Criteria

Some of the key factors that determine eligibility for a kidney transplant include:

- **End-stage renal disease (ESRD):** A kidney transplant is generally only considered for people with ESRD, which means your kidneys have lost most of their ability to function (typically with a GFR of less than 15 mL/min). People with advanced CKD who are approaching ESRD may also be evaluated for a transplant in preparation for when they need it.

- **General health:** You need to be healthy enough to undergo major surgery and tolerate the immunosuppressive medications required after a transplant. People with serious health conditions, such as advanced heart disease, cancer, or significant infections, may not be considered eligible until these conditions are managed.
- **Age:** There is no strict age limit for kidney transplants, but younger patients tend to be better candidates because they are more likely to tolerate the surgery and post-transplant care. That said, many older adults (even in their 70s or 80s) are considered eligible if they are otherwise healthy and able to handle the surgery and medications.
- **Lifestyle and ability to adhere to care:** Kidney transplant recipients need to follow a strict post-transplant regimen that includes taking immunosuppressive medications for life and attending regular follow-up appointments. Candidates who demonstrate that they can adhere to this level of care, avoid smoking, and maintain a healthy lifestyle are more likely to be eligible.
- **Psychosocial factors:** Mental health, social support, and access to resources are also evaluated. This ensures that patients have a stable support system, access to transportation for follow-up visits, and the ability to manage the emotional and physical challenges of post-transplant life.

Conditions That May Affect Eligibility

Some medical conditions can make a person ineligible for a kidney transplant or require additional management before a transplant is possible. These may include:

- **Active infections:** If you have an untreated infection or a condition that increases your risk of infection (such as HIV), you may need to manage or treat the infection before being considered for a transplant.
- **Heart disease:** Severe heart disease may disqualify some patients from transplant eligibility unless it is well-managed. Tests like echocardiograms and stress tests will help assess your heart health.
- **Obesity:** Being significantly overweight can increase the risk of complications during and after surgery. Some transplant centers may require patients to lose weight before being listed for a kidney transplant.
- **Substance use:** Active substance abuse (such as alcohol or drug use) may disqualify a candidate from a kidney transplant. Patients must demonstrate a commitment to sobriety before being considered.

The Kidney Transplant Evaluation Process

The kidney transplant evaluation is a comprehensive process designed to assess your overall health, ensure you are a good candidate for a transplant, and prepare you for life after the transplant. The evaluation typically includes:

Medical Tests and Examinations

Your healthcare team will perform a series of medical tests to determine whether you are physically capable of undergoing a transplant and if you are likely to benefit from the surgery. Some of the key tests and evaluations may include:

- **Blood tests:** Blood tests are done to assess kidney function, determine your blood type, and check for diseases such as hepatitis and HIV. Your blood type is essential for matching with a donor.
- **Heart and lung function tests:** Tests such as an electrocardiogram (ECG), echocardiogram, or stress test are conducted to evaluate your heart health and ensure your cardiovascular system can handle the surgery.
- **Cancer screenings:** Screening for certain types of cancers is important before a transplant to ensure you don't have any undiagnosed malignancies. This may include mammograms, colonoscopies, or prostate exams, depending on your age and gender.

Consultations with Specialists

During the evaluation process, you will meet with several specialists who will assess your health and provide recommendations for your care:

- **Nephrologist:** Your kidney specialist will assess your kidney disease, review your medical history, and discuss your treatment options, including dialysis if you haven't started already.
- **Transplant surgeon:** A transplant surgeon will review the risks and benefits of the surgery, explain the procedure, and assess whether you're a suitable candidate.
- **Psychologist or social worker:** Mental health professionals will evaluate your emotional readiness for the transplant, your social support system, and your ability to cope with the lifestyle changes that come with a transplant.

Psychosocial Evaluation

This part of the evaluation helps ensure that you have the necessary support and resources to manage life after a transplant. Some of the factors considered include:

- **Support system:** Do you have family, friends, or caregivers who can assist you after the transplant? A strong support system is essential for recovery and managing your post-transplant regimen.
- **Financial readiness:** The cost of a kidney transplant and ongoing medical care can be significant. A financial counselor will help you understand the costs involved and determine what your insurance covers.
- **Lifestyle:** The evaluation will also consider whether you are committed to maintaining a healthy lifestyle, including quitting smoking, avoiding alcohol or drug abuse, and adhering to dietary recommendations.

Getting on the Kidney Transplant List

If you are deemed eligible for a kidney transplant, the next step is getting on the transplant list. This process involves registering with a transplant center and waiting for a suitable donor kidney to become available.

The National Waiting List

In most countries, including the United States, kidney transplant candidates are placed on a national waiting list managed by organizations like the United Network for Organ Sharing (UNOS). The waiting list prioritizes patients based on several factors, including:

- **Blood type and compatibility:** Your blood type and tissue type must match with a donor kidney to reduce the risk of rejection. The closer the match, the better the chances of a successful transplant.

- **Time spent on dialysis:** The longer you've been on dialysis or waiting for a transplant, the higher your priority on the list.
- **Urgency:** Patients who are in more urgent need of a transplant may be prioritized, particularly if their health is deteriorating rapidly.

Living Donor Transplant

While many people receive kidneys from deceased donors, one of the best ways to shorten the waiting time and improve the chances of a successful transplant is through a living donor. A living donor can be a family member, friend, or even an altruistic donor (someone who donates without knowing the recipient).

- **Living donor advantages:** A kidney from a living donor often works better and lasts longer than a kidney from a deceased donor. Additionally, you can schedule the surgery in advance, reducing waiting times.
- **Matching process:** The living donor will undergo testing to ensure they are a match for you and that they are healthy enough to donate a kidney. The donor and recipient must have compatible blood types, and ideally, similar tissue types to reduce the risk of rejection.

What If You're Not Eligible for a Transplant?

For some people, a kidney transplant may not be an option due to medical, financial, or social reasons. If you are not eligible for a transplant, other treatments, such as dialysis, can help manage kidney failure and prolong your life. Your healthcare team will work with you to develop a comprehensive care plan that meets your needs and helps manage the symptoms of ESRD.

The Kidney Transplant Procedure

A kidney transplant is a major surgical procedure, typically performed under general anesthesia. The process involves several key steps, from preparing the patient for surgery to post-transplant care.

Preparation for Surgery

Before the transplant surgery, a series of tests and evaluations will be conducted to ensure the recipient is healthy enough to undergo the procedure. This includes blood tests, imaging studies, and assessments of heart and lung function.

- **Compatibility testing:** If a living donor has been identified, compatibility testing will be performed to ensure that the donor's kidney is a good match for the recipient. This includes checking blood type, tissue typing (HLA matching), and crossmatching (ensuring the recipient's immune system won't reject the donor kidney).

- **Deceased donor kidney:** If the transplant is from a deceased donor, the recipient will be notified when a compatible kidney becomes available, and surgery will be scheduled as quickly as possible.

During the Surgery

The kidney transplant surgery itself usually takes about 3 to 5 hours, depending on the complexity of the case.

- **Incision and placement:** The surgeon will make an incision in the lower abdomen, near the pelvis, to access the blood vessels. The new kidney is placed in this location because it provides easy access to the blood vessels and bladder.

- **Connecting the kidney:** The new kidney is connected to the recipient's blood vessels, which will allow blood to flow through the kidney and enable it to filter waste. The ureter (the tube that carries urine from the kidney to the bladder) is also connected to the bladder so that the new kidney can produce urine.
- **Monitoring function:** Once the kidney is connected, the surgical team will monitor its blood flow and ensure that it is functioning properly before closing the incision.

After the Surgery

After the surgery, the recipient will be monitored closely in the hospital for signs of kidney function, complications, or rejection.

- **Hospital stay:** Most patients remain in the hospital for several days after the transplant to ensure the new kidney is functioning and that there are no immediate complications, such as infection or blood clots.
- **Immediate function:** In some cases, the new kidney will start working immediately and produce urine right away. In other cases, especially with deceased donor kidneys, it may take a few days for the kidney to start functioning. Dialysis may be needed temporarily until the kidney starts working.

Medications After a Kidney Transplant

After a kidney transplant, the recipient will need to take several medications to help the body accept the new kidney and prevent rejection. These medications are usually taken for life and must be carefully managed to ensure the success of the transplant.

Immunosuppressive Medications

The body's immune system naturally tries to reject foreign objects, including transplanted organs. To prevent this, patients must take immunosuppressive medications (anti-rejection drugs) that weaken the immune system and stop it from attacking the new kidney.

- **Common immunosuppressive drugs:** Medications like tacrolimus (Prograf), mycophenolate mofetil (Cellcept), and prednisone are commonly prescribed to prevent rejection. These medications must be taken exactly as prescribed to maintain the delicate balance between protecting the kidney and avoiding over-suppression of the immune system.
- **Side effects:** Immunosuppressive medications can have side effects, including increased risk of infection, high blood pressure, diabetes, and weight gain. Your healthcare team will work with you to manage these side effects and ensure you stay as healthy as possible.

Other Medications

In addition to immunosuppressive drugs, patients may need to take other medications to manage blood pressure, prevent infections, and support overall health. These may include:

- Antibiotics and antiviral medications to prevent infections, particularly in the early months after the transplant when the immune system is most suppressed.
- Blood pressure medications to keep blood pressure under control and reduce the strain on the new kidney.
- Anti-ulcer medications to protect the stomach lining from the side effects of immunosuppressive drugs, which can sometimes cause gastrointestinal issues.

Risks and Complications of Kidney Transplant

While kidney transplants are generally safe and have high success rates, like any major surgery, they come with certain risks and potential complications.

- **Rejection:** The most significant risk after a transplant is organ rejection, where the body's immune system attacks the new kidney. Acute rejection can happen in the early weeks or months after the surgery, but it can also occur later. This is why taking immunosuppressive medications as prescribed is so critical. Regular monitoring through blood tests will help detect signs of rejection early so it can be treated promptly.
- **Infection:** Because immunosuppressive medications weaken the immune system, patients are more susceptible to infections, especially in the first few months after the transplant. It's important to take precautions to avoid exposure to illness and follow any infection prevention guidelines provided by your healthcare team.
- **Blood clots:** In the days following surgery, there's a risk of developing blood clots in the legs or lungs. You may be given blood thinners to reduce this risk, and early movement after surgery is encouraged to promote circulation.
- **Other complications:** Complications like bleeding, delayed kidney function, or issues related to the surgical site (such as infections or hernias) can also occur, but these are typically manageable with prompt medical care.

Long-Term Care and Monitoring

A successful kidney transplant requires lifelong management and regular check-ups to ensure the new kidney continues to function well. Your healthcare team will work closely with you to monitor your kidney function, adjust your medications, and help you maintain a healthy lifestyle.

• **Regular lab tests:** Blood tests to monitor kidney function (such as creatinine and glomerular filtration rate, or GFR) will be done frequently in the early stages after surgery and less often as you progress. These tests help detect any early signs of rejection or complications.

• **Lifestyle changes:** Maintaining a healthy lifestyle is key to keeping your new kidney functioning for as long as possible. This includes following a kidney-friendly diet, staying physically active, managing blood pressure, and avoiding smoking and excessive alcohol use.

• **Follow-up appointments:** Regular follow-up visits with your nephrologist and transplant team are essential for long-term success. These visits will ensure your medications are working effectively and that any issues are caught and addressed early.

Life After a Transplant: What Recovery Looks Like

Receiving a kidney transplant is a major life event, and the post-transplant recovery process plays a crucial role in ensuring the long-term success of the new kidney. After the surgery, your body will need time to heal, and you'll need to adjust to a new routine that includes lifelong medications, regular monitoring, and lifestyle changes. Understanding what recovery looks like after a kidney transplant can help you prepare for the physical, emotional, and practical aspects of life after surgery.

The Immediate Recovery Period

After a kidney transplant, you will spend several days to a week in the hospital under close observation. The immediate recovery period focuses on ensuring the new kidney is functioning, preventing complications, and helping your body adjust to the new organ.

Hospital Stay

- **Monitoring kidney function:** After surgery, your healthcare team will monitor your new kidney closely to make sure it's working properly. Blood tests will check levels of creatinine and other markers of kidney function. In many cases, the new kidney starts producing urine almost immediately, but in some cases, it may take a few days for the kidney to start working fully.

- **Pain management:** You will likely experience some pain or discomfort at the site of the surgery, but this can be managed with pain medications. Most patients find that the pain improves significantly within the first week.

- **Immunosuppressive medications:** To prevent your body from rejecting the new kidney, you will start taking immunosuppressive medications (anti-rejection drugs) immediately after surgery. These medications weaken your immune system so that it doesn't attack the new organ, and you'll need to continue taking them for the rest of your life.

- **Preventing infection:** Since immunosuppressive medications weaken your immune system, you'll be at a higher risk for infections, especially in the first few months after the transplant. In the hospital, you will be closely monitored for signs of infection, and you may be given antibiotics or antiviral medications to reduce this risk.

Post-Hospital Care

Once you're discharged from the hospital, your recovery will continue at home. You'll need to follow a specific care plan designed by your transplant team to ensure your new kidney remains healthy and that you avoid complications.

- **Wound care:** You'll be given instructions on how to care for the surgical site to prevent infection. Keep the area clean and dry, and watch for any signs of infection, such as redness, swelling, or drainage.
- **Follow-up appointments:** You will have frequent follow-up appointments with your transplant team in the weeks and months following your surgery. These visits are essential for monitoring kidney function, adjusting medications, and catching any signs of complications early. Initially, you may need blood tests several times a week, but as your recovery progresses, the frequency of these visits will decrease.

Medications After a Kidney Transplant

One of the most important aspects of life after a kidney transplant is taking your medications as prescribed. Immunosuppressive medications will be a part of your daily routine for the rest of your life to prevent rejection of the new kidney.

Immunosuppressive Medications (Anti-Rejection Drugs)

After a kidney transplant, your body's immune system will naturally recognize the new kidney as foreign and try to reject it. To prevent this, you will need to take immunosuppressive drugs every day to suppress your immune response and protect the new kidney.

- **Types of immunosuppressive medications:** Common immunosuppressive drugs include tacrolimus (Prograf), mycophenolate mofetil (Cellcept), and prednisone. These medications work together to prevent rejection, but they must be taken exactly as prescribed to be effective.
- **Side effects:** Immunosuppressive medications can cause side effects, including increased risk of infection, high blood pressure, weight gain, and a higher risk of certain cancers. Your healthcare team will work with you to manage these side effects and monitor your health closely.

Other Medications

In addition to immunosuppressive drugs, you may need to take other medications to manage side effects and protect your health.

- **Antibiotics and antivirals:** To prevent infections, especially during the early months after the transplant, you may be prescribed antibiotics, antiviral medications, or antifungal medications.
- **Blood pressure medications:** Many people who receive a kidney transplant still need to take medications to control their blood pressure, even if their new kidney is functioning well.
- **Medications for blood sugar:** Immunosuppressive medications, particularly steroids like prednisone, can cause blood sugar levels to rise. You may need to take medications to manage blood sugar, especially if you develop diabetes after the transplant.

Adjusting to Life After a Transplant

While life after a kidney transplant can offer a much greater quality of life compared to dialysis, it requires some adjustments. Establishing a new routine that includes medications, regular monitoring, and lifestyle changes will be key to your long-term health.

Dietary Changes

After a kidney transplant, your diet will likely change, and you'll need to follow certain guidelines to keep your new kidney functioning well.

- **Balanced diet:** Your dietitian will help you develop a balanced diet that provides the nutrients you need to stay healthy. You may no longer need the strict restrictions required for CKD or dialysis, but you'll still need to be mindful of certain nutrients like sodium and fats to protect your new kidney and prevent complications.
- **Limit certain foods:** While you may have more freedom in your diet, it's important to avoid certain foods that can increase your risk of infection. These may include raw or undercooked meats, unpasteurized dairy products, and certain types of raw fish like sushi.

Exercise and Physical Activity

Staying physically active is an important part of your recovery and long-term health after a kidney transplant. Regular exercise can help you regain strength, improve cardiovascular health, and maintain a healthy weight.

- **Start slowly:** In the first few weeks after surgery, your physical activity will be limited as your body heals. Start with light activities like walking, and gradually increase your activity level as recommended by your doctor.

- **Build a routine:** Once you've recovered from the surgery, aim to incorporate regular exercise into your routine. Activities like walking, swimming, and cycling are great for maintaining your fitness and overall health.

Emotional and Mental Health

Receiving a kidney transplant is a significant emotional and mental adjustment. While many people feel relief and optimism after the surgery, it's also normal to experience anxiety or uncertainty as you adapt to your new life.

- **Seek support:** It's important to have a strong support system in place. Talk to family, friends, or counselors about any feelings of anxiety, stress, or depression you may experience during your recovery.

- **Join a support group:** Many people find comfort in connecting with others who have undergone kidney transplants. Support groups can offer valuable advice, encouragement, and a sense of community as you navigate life after surgery.

Long-Term Care and Monitoring

A successful kidney transplant requires lifelong monitoring and care to ensure the new kidney continues to function well. Your healthcare team will provide regular check-ups and blood tests to monitor kidney function, detect signs of rejection early, and adjust medications as needed.

Routine Blood Tests and Follow-Up

After your transplant, you will have regular blood tests to monitor how well your new kidney is working. These tests will measure levels of creatinine, blood urea nitrogen (BUN), and other markers of kidney function.

- **Frequent tests initially:** In the early months after the transplant, blood tests may be needed several times a week. As you recover and the new kidney stabilizes, the frequency of these tests will decrease.
- **Long-term follow-up:** Even years after the transplant, regular check-ups are essential to monitor for signs of rejection or complications. Ongoing follow-up care is critical for maintaining your health and extending the life of your new kidney.

Signs of Rejection

Although the risk of rejection decreases over time, it's still possible for the body to reject the new kidney months or even years after the transplant. It's important to recognize the signs of rejection so that prompt treatment can be started if needed.

- **Symptoms of rejection:** Signs of rejection may include fever, decreased urine output, swelling in the legs or ankles, sudden weight gain, or pain over the kidney area. If you notice any of these symptoms, contact your healthcare provider immediately.

The Benefits of a Kidney Transplant

While the post-transplant period involves careful management and lifestyle changes, a kidney transplant offers significant benefits compared to dialysis, including:

- **Improved quality of life:** Many people report feeling more energetic and physically active after a successful transplant. You may have fewer dietary and fluid restrictions, and you won't need to spend hours on dialysis.
- **Increased life expectancy:** For most people, a kidney transplant can significantly extend life expectancy compared to remaining on dialysis. A successful transplant can last for many years, and some people live with a transplanted kidney for decades.

CHAPTER EIGHT

LONG-TERM MANAGEMENT OF CKD

Regular Check-Ups and Monitoring

The Importance of Tracking Kidney Function with Blood and Urine Tests

For people living with Chronic Kidney Disease (CKD), regular monitoring of kidney function is vital to assess how well the kidneys are working and to detect any changes in the progression of the disease. Blood and urine tests provide important insights into your kidney health and guide decisions about your treatment plan. These tests help your healthcare team identify potential complications early and adjust medications, lifestyle recommendations, or therapies to better manage your condition.

This section will explore why blood and urine tests are essential for tracking kidney function and what these tests reveal about your kidney health.

Key Blood Tests for Monitoring Kidney Function

Blood tests are one of the most reliable ways to measure kidney function and detect changes in how well your kidneys are filtering waste from your blood. Below are the most common blood tests used to monitor kidney health in people with CKD.

CREATININE LEVELS

Creatinine is a waste product produced by muscle metabolism and excreted by the kidneys. It's one of the most important markers of kidney function because healthy kidneys filter creatinine from the blood. When your kidneys aren't working properly, creatinine builds up in the bloodstream.

High creatinine levels: Elevated creatinine levels in the blood are a sign that your kidneys are not filtering waste as effectively as they should. As CKD progresses, creatinine levels typically rise, indicating worsening kidney function. Normal ranges: For most adults, normal creatinine levels are between 0.6 to 1.2 mg/dL for men and 0.5 to 1.1 mg/dL for women. Your doctor will compare your current creatinine levels with previous tests to track any changes in kidney function.

GLOMERULAR FILTRATION RATE (GFR)

The Glomerular Filtration Rate (GFR) is a calculation that estimates how well your kidneys are filtering waste from the blood. It is considered one of the most accurate measures of kidney function and is calculated based on your creatinine levels, age, gender, and race.

Stages of CKD based on GFR:

Stage 1 CKD: GFR of 90 mL/min or higher (normal or near normal kidney function with signs of kidney damage)
Stage 2 CKD: GFR between 60 and 89 mL/min (mild loss of kidney function)
Stage 3 CKD: GFR between 30 and 59 mL/min (moderate loss of kidney function)
Stage 4 CKD: GFR between 15 and 29 mL/min (severe loss of kidney function)
Stage 5 CKD: GFR less than 15 mL/min (kidney failure or end-stage renal disease)
Tracking GFR over time: Your GFR will be monitored regularly to track the progression of CKD. A decreasing GFR indicates a decline in kidney function, while a stable or improving GFR suggests that treatment is working to slow disease progression.

Blood Urea Nitrogen (BUN)

Blood Urea Nitrogen (BUN) is another waste product that the kidneys filter out of the blood. Like creatinine, BUN levels rise when kidney function declines.

High BUN levels: Elevated BUN levels indicate that your kidneys are not filtering waste effectively, which can be a sign of worsening CKD.

Normal ranges: Normal BUN levels typically range between 7 and 20 mg/dL. Your healthcare provider will monitor these levels alongside creatinine and GFR to assess kidney function.

ELECTROLYTE LEVELS

CKD can affect your body's balance of electrolytes, such as potassium, sodium, and calcium. Blood tests will measure these electrolytes to ensure they remain within a healthy range.

Potassium: High levels of potassium (hyperkalemia) can be dangerous and may cause heart problems, so it's important to monitor potassium levels closely. If your kidneys are not filtering potassium effectively, your doctor may recommend dietary changes or medications to manage potassium levels.
Sodium: Low sodium levels (hyponatremia) can result from fluid retention, which is common in CKD. Your doctor will monitor sodium levels and may recommend adjustments to your fluid intake if needed.
Calcium and phosphorus: Kidney disease can affect the balance of calcium and phosphorus, leading to bone problems. Blood tests will track these levels to ensure your bones stay healthy and to prevent complications like chronic kidney disease-mineral and bone disorder (CKD-MBD).

Key Urine Tests for Monitoring Kidney Function

Urine tests are another important tool for evaluating kidney function and detecting signs of kidney damage. These tests can reveal how well your kidneys are filtering waste and whether there is any protein or blood in your urine, which are signs of kidney damage.

URINE ALBUMIN-TO-CREATININE RATIO (ACR)

One of the earliest signs of kidney damage is the presence of albumin, a type of protein, in your urine. Healthy kidneys typically prevent protein from passing into the urine, but damaged kidneys may allow it to leak through.

Proteinuria (albumin in the urine): The presence of albumin in the urine is called proteinuria. Proteinuria is a common sign of kidney damage and can occur in the early stages of CKD, even before there is a significant decline in kidney function.

ALBUMIN-TO-CREATININE RATIO (ACR): The ACR test measures the amount of albumin in your urine compared to the amount of creatinine. This provides an accurate indication of whether your kidneys are leaking protein. An ACR of 30 mg/g or higher is considered abnormal and may indicate kidney damage.

24-Hour Urine Test

In some cases, your doctor may ask you to collect your urine over a 24-hour period to get a more accurate picture of how well your kidneys are working. This test measures the total amount of urine your kidneys produce and can provide additional information about kidney function and electrolyte balance.

Measuring urine output: A 24-hour urine collection can reveal how much urine your kidneys are producing, which is important for assessing fluid balance and kidney function.

Electrolyte excretion: This test can also measure how much sodium, potassium, calcium, and other electrolytes your kidneys are excreting, helping your doctor make adjustments to your diet or medications if needed.

How Often Should Kidney Function Be Monitored?

The frequency of blood and urine tests will depend on the stage of your CKD and your overall health. In the early stages of CKD, tests may be done every few months, while more advanced stages may require more frequent monitoring.
Early stages (Stage 1-3 CKD): If your kidney function is relatively stable, your doctor may recommend testing every 3 to 6 months to track any changes in kidney function.
Later stages (Stage 4-5 CKD): As CKD progresses, more frequent monitoring (every 1 to 3 months) may be necessary to detect any worsening of kidney function and manage complications like anemia, electrolyte imbalances, or bone disease.
Dialysis or transplant: If you are on dialysis or have had a kidney transplant, even more frequent monitoring may be required to ensure your treatment is working and to catch any signs of complications early.

How to Stay on Top of Your Health with Doctor Visits and Routine Tests

Staying proactive with your health is essential when managing Chronic Kidney Disease (CKD). Regular doctor visits and routine tests allow for ongoing assessment of kidney function and help detect potential complications early. By closely monitoring your condition, you and your healthcare team can make timely adjustments to your treatment plan and slow the progression of the disease. Being organized and involved in your care can also help reduce anxiety and ensure that you're staying on top of your overall health.

In this section, we'll discuss practical tips on how to stay on track with your doctor visits and routine tests, and how you can actively participate in managing your CKD.

1. Scheduling and Preparing for Doctor Visits

One of the best ways to stay on top of your health is by regularly scheduling and attending doctor visits. Your nephrologist will be your main partner in managing CKD, but you may also need to visit other specialists, such as a cardiologist or dietitian, depending on your needs.

Keep Track of Appointments

It's important to have a system in place to keep track of your upcoming appointments and tests. Missing appointments or delaying tests can lead to gaps in your care and make it harder to manage your condition effectively.

- **Use a calendar:** Whether you prefer a paper calendar, a digital planner, or a smartphone app, make sure to mark down all of your medical appointments, follow-up tests, and any other related events. Set reminders a few days before each appointment so you don't miss anything.

- **Plan in advance:** Schedule your next appointment before you leave your doctor's office, or make a note to call ahead to book the appointment. This helps prevent gaps in your care and ensures that you stay on a regular schedule.

Prepare Questions Ahead of Time

Doctor visits are a valuable opportunity to ask questions, clarify your treatment plan, and discuss any new symptoms or concerns. Preparing a list of questions ahead of time can help you make the most of your visit.

Common questions to ask: Consider asking about the results of your most recent tests, changes in your medication, how your CKD is progressing, and what steps you can take to improve your kidney health. If you've noticed new symptoms or side effects from medications, make sure to bring them up during your visit.

Bring a support person: If possible, bring a family member or friend with you to appointments. They can help take notes, ask additional questions, and provide emotional support. It can also be helpful to have someone else who understands your condition and can assist with managing your care.

2. Following Up on Routine Tests

Routine blood and urine tests are critical for tracking CKD progression. It's important to follow through on scheduled tests and stay informed about your results. These tests help your doctor adjust your treatment plan based on real-time data about your kidney function and overall health.

Know When Your Tests Are Due

Your doctor will provide a schedule for routine tests, which may vary depending on the stage of your CKD. Knowing when your next test is due helps ensure you stay on track with your care.

Stick to the schedule: Missing or delaying tests can lead to inaccurate assessments of your kidney health. Make sure to schedule lab appointments well in advance, and set reminders for yourself.

Ask about new tests: As your condition changes, your doctor may recommend additional tests to monitor complications like anemia, electrolyte imbalances, or bone health. Don't hesitate to ask your healthcare provider if any new tests are necessary to assess your condition more thoroughly.

Understand Your Test Results

It's important to understand the significance of your test results so that you can actively participate in your care. If you don't understand something about your results, ask your healthcare provider to explain them in simpler terms.

Track key markers: Pay attention to important indicators of kidney health, such as GFR, creatinine, BUN, and albumin levels. By knowing your baseline numbers and how they change over time, you'll be more empowered to engage in your care and make informed decisions.

Use a patient portal: Many healthcare providers offer online patient portals where you can view your test results, communicate with your doctor, and schedule appointments.

Take advantage of this technology to stay on top of your health data and follow up on any concerns promptly.

3. Staying Organized with Your Health Information

Organizing your health information can help you keep track of your medical history, medications, and test results. Being organized also makes it easier to share information with your healthcare team and stay on top of your care.

Create a Medical File

Keep a physical or digital folder that includes all of your medical records, test results, medication lists, and doctor's notes. This file should be easily accessible and kept up to date.

Medical history: Include a summary of your medical history, including the diagnosis of CKD, any other conditions you have, and surgeries or treatments you've undergone.

Medications: Keep an up-to-date list of all the medications you are taking, including dosages, frequency, and any side effects you've noticed. This is particularly important if you're seeing multiple specialists or starting new treatments.

Use a Health App

There are many health-tracking apps available that allow you to record your medications, track your symptoms, and store your medical information. Some apps can even send you reminders about upcoming appointments or tests.

Track your progress: Using a health app, you can track your blood pressure, weight, or any other symptoms you're monitoring as part of your CKD management. This data can help your doctor assess your progress and make adjustments to your treatment plan.

Set medication reminders: Some apps allow you to set reminders to take your medications on time, which is especially helpful for managing complex medication regimens, such as those that include multiple doses or require special timing.

4. Communicating with Your Healthcare Team

Clear and consistent communication with your healthcare team is essential for managing CKD effectively. If you have questions about your treatment plan, symptoms, or test results, don't hesitate to reach out to your doctor or nurse.

Ask About Your Treatment Plan

If you're unsure about any part of your treatment plan—whether it's how to take a new medication, how to prepare for a test, or how to follow dietary recommendations—ask your healthcare provider for clarification.

Stay involved in decision-making: Your healthcare team will work with you to create a treatment plan that fits your needs and preferences. Make sure you understand the goals of each part of the plan and provide input on what works best for your lifestyle.

Follow up on any changes: If your doctor makes changes to your medications, diet, or exercise plan, schedule a follow-up appointment to discuss how these changes are working. If something isn't working, your healthcare team can make adjustments to better suit your needs.

Keep Your Doctor Informed of Changes

If you notice any new symptoms, changes in your condition, or side effects from your medications, it's important to inform your healthcare provider as soon as possible.

Report new symptoms: Common CKD symptoms like fatigue, swelling, or changes in urination should be reported to your doctor right away, especially if they worsen or are accompanied by other problems like nausea or dizziness. **Discuss side effects:** Some medications used to manage CKD, such as blood pressure medications or phosphate binders, may cause side effects. Let your doctor know if you're experiencing any side effects so they can adjust your medications or suggest alternatives.

Keeping a Healthy Routine

Creating a Daily Schedule that Supports Kidney Health

Living with Chronic Kidney Disease (CKD) requires consistent attention to lifestyle habits and medical care. Creating a daily schedule that prioritizes kidney health can help you stay organized and make better decisions about your diet, exercise, medications, and overall well-being. A structured routine ensures you meet your health goals, take medications on time, and integrate healthy habits into your everyday life.

Setting priorities for your daily routine is essential when living with CKD. The most important areas to focus on include medication management, adhering to a kidney-friendly diet, staying active, and ensuring you get enough rest and hydration. These are the pillars of your daily routine, and you can shape your schedule around them.

Start by organizing your medication schedule. Many people with CKD need to take medicines to control blood pressure, manage fluid balance, treat anemia, or protect kidney function. Make sure you have a reliable way to remember your medications, whether it's setting alarms on your phone, using a pill organizer, or creating a chart with your doses and times. Coordinating your medications with meals can also help you stay on track, as some need to be taken with food. Incorporate these times into your regular meal schedule to ensure you're consistent.

Planning your meals ahead of time is a vital part of managing CKD. Depending on your stage of CKD, your doctor or dietitian will recommend dietary guidelines to follow, such as reducing sodium, potassium, phosphorus, and protein. It's a good idea to spend time each week planning your meals to ensure they meet your dietary needs and avoid foods that could strain your kidneys. Preparing meals in advance can also help you stick to your plan, giving you healthy, ready-to-eat options that fit your diet.

Physical activity is equally important. Staying active helps manage weight, lower blood pressure, and reduce stress. Choose a specific time each day to exercise, whether it's going for a walk in the morning, doing a yoga session after lunch, or engaging in a light workout in the evening. Consistency is key, but if dedicated exercise time is hard to find, try to incorporate more movement into your day by taking short walks during breaks or doing simple stretches while watching TV. Exercise doesn't have to be strenuous; even 30 minutes of moderate activity can make a significant difference.

Prioritize rest and sleep, as they play a crucial role in your overall well-being. People with CKD often experience fatigue, so it's essential to get enough rest to help your body recover and maintain energy. Establish a consistent sleep routine by going to bed and waking up at the same time every day. Avoid stimulating activities like watching TV or using your phone an hour before bed, and instead, focus on calming activities such as reading or light stretching to wind down. Managing stress throughout the day is also important for kidney health. Chronic stress can negatively impact CKD by raising blood pressure and increasing inflammation. Incorporating stress-relief practices like mindfulness, meditation, or deep breathing into your daily routine can make a significant difference in how you feel. Even short breaks for relaxation during a busy day can help manage stress levels.

Here's a sample daily schedule that could help you stay on top of your kidney health. Adjust it to fit your personal needs and lifestyle:

- Start your day at 7:00 AM with your morning medications, followed by a kidney-friendly breakfast at 7:30 AM. At 8:00 AM, take a 20-30 minute walk or do some light exercise to get your body moving. By 9:00 AM, begin your work or daily activities, but remember to take breaks and move around every hour.

- Around noon, have a kidney-friendly lunch and follow it up with a few minutes of relaxation or mindfulness. After lunch, you can resume your work or activities for the afternoon. At 3:30 PM, enjoy a healthy snack and fit in some light physical activity, like stretching or a brief walk.

- Dinner around 6:00 PM should be balanced and fit your dietary requirements. Afterward, take your evening medications, then spend time relaxing with activities that help you unwind. By 9:00 PM, begin your pre-bedtime routine to prepare for a good night's sleep, with the goal of getting to bed by 10:00 PM.

Adjusting your schedule based on your needs is important. If you feel fatigued, it's essential to listen to your body and rest. As your CKD progresses or your treatment plan changes, your routine may need to shift to accommodate new medications or lifestyle adjustments. Staying organized by using a planner, calendar, or health app can make it easier to keep track of medications, meal plans, and appointments. Support from family, friends, or caregivers can also make a significant difference in maintaining a healthy lifestyle.

Staying Active, Eating Well, and Reducing Stress for Long-Term Health

When managing Chronic Kidney Disease (CKD), staying active, eating a kidney-friendly diet, and effectively managing stress are three critical components to maintaining your overall health and slowing the progression of the disease. These lifestyle habits help to control complications like high blood pressure, blood sugar levels, and inflammation, all of which can negatively impact kidney function if left unchecked. This section will explore the importance of physical activity, nutrition, and stress reduction, offering practical steps to incorporate these habits into your daily routine for long-term kidney health.

Staying Active
Physical activity is beneficial for everyone, but for people with CKD, it can play a vital role in maintaining cardiovascular health, managing weight, and reducing stress. Regular exercise helps improve circulation, strengthen the heart, and keep blood pressure in check, all of which are essential for protecting kidney function. Additionally, exercise helps boost energy levels, reduces feelings of fatigue, and promotes emotional well-being by releasing endorphins—natural mood enhancers.
If you're new to exercise or haven't been active for a while, it's important to start slow and gradually increase your level of physical activity. Even simple activities like walking, swimming, or yoga can have significant benefits. Aim to incorporate at least 30 minutes of moderate-intensity exercise

into your routine most days of the week. You can break it up into shorter sessions throughout the day if needed, such as taking a 10-minute walk after each meal.

Strength training, using light weights or resistance bands, can also help maintain muscle mass and improve strength, which can be particularly important for people with CKD, as muscle loss can be a concern. Flexibility exercises like stretching or yoga are useful for maintaining joint health and mobility, reducing stiffness, and promoting relaxation. Always consult your healthcare provider before starting a new exercise regimen, especially if you have any other medical conditions.

Eating Well

Nutrition plays a pivotal role in managing CKD. A kidney-friendly diet can help prevent further damage to your kidneys, manage symptoms, and reduce the risk of complications like high blood pressure, electrolyte imbalances, and bone disease. Depending on the stage of your CKD, you may need to follow specific dietary restrictions to limit certain nutrients, such as sodium, potassium, phosphorus, and protein.

One of the most important aspects of a kidney-friendly diet is limiting sodium. High sodium intake can lead to fluid retention, swelling, and increased blood pressure, all of which can strain the kidneys. Aim to consume less than 2,000 milligrams of sodium per day by avoiding processed and packaged foods, which often contain hidden salt. Instead, season your food with herbs, spices, and natural flavorings like lemon or vinegar to reduce your sodium intake without sacrificing flavor.

Potassium and phosphorus are two other nutrients that may need to be limited, particularly in the later stages of CKD. High potassium levels (hyperkalemia) can lead to heart problems, while excess phosphorus can weaken your bones. Your doctor or dietitian will guide you on how to manage these nutrients based on your individual needs. Foods rich in potassium include bananas, oranges, potatoes, and tomatoes, while phosphorus is often found in dairy products, nuts, seeds, and certain types of meat. You may also need to adjust your protein intake. While protein is important for maintaining muscle mass, too much protein can produce waste products that are hard for the kidneys to filter. Depending on your condition, your dietitian may recommend limiting protein or focusing on high-quality protein sources, such as lean meats, fish, eggs, or plant-based proteins like tofu.

Hydration is another key factor in managing CKD. Your healthcare provider will advise you on how much fluid to drink based on your kidney function and stage of CKD. Staying hydrated is important, but overconsumption of fluids can cause complications like swelling or high blood pressure, especially for those in the later stages of CKD.

Reducing Stress

Stress management is critical for people with CKD, as chronic stress can exacerbate symptoms and increase the risk of complications like high blood pressure. Stress triggers the release of hormones that can raise blood pressure and heart rate, putting additional strain on your kidneys. By incorporating relaxation techniques and mindfulness practices into your daily routine, you can help reduce stress and protect your kidney health.

Mindfulness meditation is a highly effective way to manage stress and promote emotional well-being. Taking just a few minutes each day to focus on your breathing and bring your attention to the present moment can help calm your mind and lower stress levels. Deep breathing exercises are another simple and effective way to reduce stress. Practice taking slow, deep breaths for a few minutes whenever you feel overwhelmed or anxious. This helps activate your body's relaxation response, lowering your heart rate and blood pressure.

Physical activity can also be a powerful stress reliever. Regular exercise releases endorphins, which are natural mood boosters, and helps reduce the physical tension that builds up in your body when you're stressed. Activities like yoga, tai chi, or even a brisk walk can have both physical and mental health benefits by combining movement with mindful relaxation.

Another helpful strategy for reducing stress is to build a strong support network. Connecting with family, friends, or a support group can provide emotional support and encouragement, making it easier to cope with the challenges of managing CKD. Don't hesitate to reach out to others when you need help, whether it's to talk about how you're feeling or to share practical tips on managing the disease.

Staying Informed About New Treatments

Talking to Your Doctor About New Medications and Therapies

As new medications and therapies for Chronic Kidney Disease (CKD) continue to emerge, it's important to have open and informed discussions with your doctor about these advancements. Introducing new treatments to your care plan can be complex, and making sure these therapies are safe and effective for your specific condition is essential. By understanding the latest options and discussing them with your healthcare provider, you can ensure that you're receiving the best possible care.

When you hear about a new medication, therapy, or clinical trial that might benefit your CKD treatment, it's important to bring it up during your next visit to your healthcare provider. Your doctor can explain how the new treatment works, whether it's appropriate for your condition, and what the potential risks and benefits might be.

It's important to ask your doctor if a new medication is suitable for your stage of CKD. Different stages of CKD require different treatment approaches, and what may work for someone else might not be appropriate for you. Your doctor will also evaluate how the new treatment compares to your current medications and whether it could offer any additional benefits.

When discussing new treatments, you need to evaluate the potential benefits and risks. Every medication has the potential for side effects, so it's crucial to understand what these are. Your doctor will help you weigh the expected improvements in your condition against any possible side effects or risks.

Introducing a new therapy may also affect other aspects of your treatment plan. Your doctor can explain whether the new medication will replace or add to your current regimen and if any changes to your routine will be necessary.

If you're interested in participating in a clinical trial, your doctor can help you assess whether you're eligible. Clinical trials can offer access to experimental treatments that aren't yet widely available, but there are usually strict eligibility criteria based on your health and stage of CKD. Your doctor will review these criteria and explain what benefits the trial might offer you.

It's essential to understand the commitment required for a clinical trial, as it often involves additional monitoring, frequent visits, and tests. Before enrolling, ensure you're aware of all the procedures involved and how they might impact your daily life. Clinical trials are closely monitored to ensure participant safety, and your doctor will help you assess the risks associated with participating. If you do experience side effects during the trial, you will receive appropriate care and support.

Even if you're not pursuing new treatments at the moment, it's crucial to stay engaged with your ongoing care. CKD is a progressive disease, and your treatment plan may need adjustments as your condition evolves. Regular check-ups allow your doctor to monitor your kidney function and make necessary changes to keep your CKD under control.

Your doctor can provide you with updates on any new research or developments in CKD treatments, even if your current plan is working well. Staying informed ensures that you have access to the best available options for managing your condition.

Proactively managing CKD is key to preventing complications and slowing disease progression. Make sure to follow your doctor's recommendations on medications, diet, and lifestyle changes. Staying consistent with your treatment plan helps you maintain your health and quality of life. If you have any concerns or notice changes in your condition, don't hesitate to contact your healthcare provider. Open communication is critical to ensuring you receive the best possible care.

Understanding the Benefits and Risks of New Medications

Each new medication or therapy for CKD comes with its own set of potential benefits and risks. Before starting any new treatment, it's important to fully understand how it may impact your kidney health, overall well-being, and current treatment plan. Your doctor will assess the effectiveness of the new medication based on clinical studies, your medical history, and how well it aligns with your needs.

When discussing new medications with your doctor, ask questions about how the treatment works, what the potential side effects are, and how it could improve your condition. Some important questions to consider include:

How does this medication or therapy work to manage CKD?

a. What are the possible side effects or risks associated with it?
b. Will it interact with my current medications or supplements?
c. How long will it take to see results, and what should I expect during that time?
d. Are there any lifestyle adjustments I need to make if I start this treatment?

Your doctor can provide answers to these questions and help weigh the pros and cons of adding a new medication or therapy to your regimen. In some cases, new treatments may offer significant improvements in managing complications like high blood pressure, anemia, or fluid retention.

However, it's important to carefully consider the risks of potential side effects or interactions with other medications you may be taking.

Staying Informed About New Therapies

As new medications and therapies for CKD are developed, it can be beneficial to stay informed about the latest research and advancements. This not only empowers you to have more meaningful conversations with your healthcare provider, but it also helps you stay proactive in your treatment.

Ask your doctor about reputable sources for staying up to date on CKD treatments, such as medical journals, trusted websites, or patient support groups. Many organizations, including the National Kidney Foundation and other health institutions, provide reliable information on emerging therapies, clinical trials, and treatment updates. By staying informed, you'll be better equipped to discuss new options with your healthcare team and make informed decisions about your care.

If you're interested in learning about potential clinical trials, your doctor can help guide you through the process of finding trials that may be appropriate for your condition. Participating in clinical trials can offer early access to new treatments, but it's essential to fully understand the trial's purpose, risks, and potential outcomes before enrolling.

Advocating for Your Kidney Health

Managing CKD requires a collaborative approach between you and your healthcare team. Being an advocate for your kidney health means taking an active role in your treatment decisions and ensuring that your concerns are addressed. If you feel that your current treatment plan isn't as effective as it could be or if you're experiencing side effects from your medications, bring these concerns to your doctor's attention. During your appointments, it's important to communicate openly about how you're feeling and how well you think your current medications are working. If you believe that a new therapy could benefit your condition, discuss this with your doctor and ask whether it's appropriate to consider a change in your treatment plan.

For example, if you're managing symptoms like fatigue, swelling, or anemia, and you've heard about new therapies that might target these specific issues, bring this information to your doctor. Together, you can evaluate whether incorporating a new treatment could improve your symptoms or overall quality of life.

Regularly Reviewing Your Treatment Plan
As CKD progresses, your treatment needs may change. Medications that were effective in earlier stages of the disease may need to be adjusted as your kidney function declines. It's essential to regularly review your treatment plan with your doctor to ensure that it continues to meet your needs and that any new therapies are considered if they become available.

At each appointment, review the effectiveness of your current medications and discuss whether there are any new therapies that could benefit you. Keep track of how you're feeling, any changes in your symptoms, and any side effects you've noticed. This information will help your doctor make informed decisions about your care.

Regularly updating your treatment plan ensures that you're receiving the most effective therapies for your stage of CKD and can help you stay on track with managing your condition.

CHAPTER NINE

LONG-TERM MANAGEMENT OF CKD

Coping with the Emotional Impact of CKD

How to Deal with Anxiety, Depression, and Fear About Your Diagnosis

Receiving a diagnosis of Chronic Kidney Disease (CKD) can trigger a wide range of emotions, including anxiety, depression, fear, and uncertainty about the future. It's normal to feel overwhelmed when you first learn about the condition and the changes it may bring to your life. Dealing with the emotional impact of CKD is just as important as managing the physical aspects, and addressing your mental health can significantly improve your quality of life. Understanding these emotions, recognizing when they are becoming overwhelming, and knowing how to seek help can make the journey with CKD more manageable.

1. Understanding the Emotional Impact of CKD

It's natural to experience anxiety and fear when faced with a chronic illness like CKD. Many people worry about how the disease will affect their day-to-day life, work, relationships, and long-term health. You might feel anxious about the need for lifestyle changes, such as dietary restrictions, medications, or possible treatments like dialysis or a kidney transplant. Depression is also common among people with CKD. The feeling of losing control over your health and future can be daunting, leading to sadness, hopelessness, or even anger. You may feel frustrated about your physical limitations, worried about the progression of the disease, or distressed about how it will impact your family and loved ones. These feelings can sometimes lead to a withdrawal from social activities or an overwhelming sense of fatigue, making it difficult to cope with daily life.

2. Recognizing Symptoms of Anxiety and Depression

While it's normal to feel worried or sad at times, prolonged or intense feelings of anxiety and depression can interfere with your ability to manage CKD effectively. Recognizing the symptoms of these mental health conditions is crucial for getting the support you need.

Common symptoms of anxiety include constant worry, difficulty concentrating, restlessness, irritability, and physical symptoms like rapid heart rate, sweating, or trouble sleeping. Anxiety may manifest as fear of the unknown or an overwhelming sense of dread about the future, especially when thinking about the progression of CKD or potential treatments like dialysis.

Depression can manifest as persistent sadness, feelings of hopelessness, loss of interest in activities you once enjoyed, changes in appetite or weight, fatigue, and difficulty sleeping. People with depression may also feel worthless or guilty, believing they are a burden to their loved ones. In more severe cases, depression can lead to thoughts of self-harm or suicide.

If you notice any of these symptoms lasting for more than a couple of weeks, it's important to speak with your doctor or a mental health professional. Addressing these feelings early can prevent them from worsening and improve your ability to manage your CKD.

3. Coping Strategies for Managing Anxiety and Depression

While dealing with anxiety and depression can feel overwhelming, there are many strategies you can use to cope with these emotions and regain a sense of control over your life.

One of the most effective ways to manage anxiety and depression is to acknowledge your feelings and understand that they are a natural response to a difficult situation. It's okay to feel scared or sad about your diagnosis. Giving yourself permission to experience these emotions without judgment can relieve some of the pressure you may be feeling.

Establishing a routine can also help manage anxiety. The unpredictability of chronic illness can make you feel like you're constantly losing control. Creating a structured daily schedule that includes time for meals, medications, exercise, and relaxation can bring a sense of normalcy to your life.

Knowing what to expect each day can reduce feelings of uncertainty and anxiety.

Engaging in mindfulness practices like meditation, deep breathing exercises, or yoga can help calm your mind and reduce stress. Mindfulness teaches you to focus on the present moment, letting go of worries about the future or regrets about the past. Even just a few minutes of mindfulness each day can help alleviate anxiety and improve your mood.
For those struggling with depression, physical activity can be a powerful mood booster. Exercise releases endorphins, which are natural chemicals in your brain that improve your mood and energy levels. You don't need to engage in strenuous workouts—simple activities like walking, swimming, or gentle stretching can make a big difference in how you feel.

Another helpful strategy is to stay connected with your support system. Isolation can worsen feelings of anxiety and depression, so it's important to reach out to friends, family, or support groups. Talking about your feelings with people who care about you can provide emotional relief and help you feel less alone. You may also want to join a CKD support group where you can connect with others who are going through similar experiences.

4. Seeking Professional Help
If you find that your anxiety or depression is interfering with your ability to manage your CKD or enjoy your life, it may be time to seek professional help. Mental health counseling or therapy can be incredibly beneficial for people dealing with

chronic illness. A therapist can help you explore your feelings, develop coping strategies, and work through fears about your diagnosis.

Cognitive Behavioral Therapy (CBT) is one type of therapy that is particularly effective for managing anxiety and depression. CBT focuses on identifying and changing negative thought patterns that contribute to feelings of anxiety or hopelessness. Through CBT, you can learn to challenge unhelpful thoughts and replace them with more balanced, realistic perspectives.

In some cases, your doctor or therapist may recommend medication to help manage severe anxiety or depression. Medications like antidepressants or anti-anxiety drugs can be a helpful tool in managing these conditions, especially when used alongside therapy or other coping strategies. Always discuss the risks and benefits of these medications with your doctor to ensure they are appropriate for your situation.

5. Taking Care of Your Emotional Well-Being
Managing your emotional health is just as important as managing your physical health when living with CKD. By acknowledging your feelings, developing healthy coping strategies, and seeking support from loved ones or professionals, you can improve your emotional well-being and strengthen your ability to cope with the challenges of CKD.

Finding Emotional Support from Family, Friends, and Support Groups

Living with Chronic Kidney Disease (CKD) can be emotionally challenging, and finding support from those around you is essential for maintaining your mental and emotional well-being. While it's natural to feel isolated at times, reaching out to family, friends, and support groups can provide a strong foundation for emotional stability. Having a support system in place helps you process your feelings, cope with the demands of managing CKD, and face the future with a greater sense of control and confidence.

This section explores the importance of seeking emotional support, how to build a strong support system, and where to find help in both local communities and online.

1. The Importance of Seeking Emotional Support

Dealing with the emotional impact of CKD can feel overwhelming, but you don't have to face it alone. Emotional support is a crucial part of managing chronic illness because it provides a space where you can express your feelings, share your concerns, and receive encouragement from others. Connecting with people who care about you can help you process complex emotions like fear, sadness, or frustration, which are common for people living with CKD.

Family and friends often want to help but may not know the best way to offer support. By opening up to them, you allow them to understand what you're going through and how they can assist. It's important to communicate your emotional needs, whether that's asking someone to listen, offering practical help with daily tasks, or simply spending time together to take your mind off your diagnosis.

In addition to leaning on loved ones, connecting with others who are going through a similar experience can provide a sense of validation and belonging. Support groups, both in-person and online, can offer a safe space to share your journey with others who truly understand the challenges of living with CKD.

2. Building a Support System

A strong support system doesn't have to consist of many people—it's about having a few key individuals or resources you can turn to when you need emotional or practical help. To build a support system that works for you, start by identifying the people in your life who are empathetic, trustworthy, and reliable.

Begin by talking to close family members or friends about your diagnosis and how it makes you feel. These initial conversations can sometimes be difficult, especially if you're unsure how they will react. However, expressing your emotions openly can help them understand your needs and give them the opportunity to offer support. For instance, you might tell a close friend, "I'm feeling overwhelmed by my CKD diagnosis, and it would really help if I could talk to you about it sometimes."

Once you've opened the conversation, don't hesitate to ask for specific kinds of support. Some people may not know how to help, so letting them know what you need can make things clearer. Whether you need someone to help with errands, join you at a doctor's appointment, or simply spend time with you, being direct about what you need can make it easier for others to step in.

In addition to family and friends, it's beneficial to connect with others who are navigating CKD. This is where support groups, both local and online, can play a pivotal role.

3. Finding Support Groups for CKD Patients
Support groups provide a valuable resource for people living with CKD, offering a community of individuals who understand the emotional and physical challenges that come with the condition. Being part of a support group allows you to share experiences, ask questions, and receive encouragement from others who are going through similar situations. Many people find that hearing about the experiences of others helps them feel less isolated and more empowered to manage their condition.

There are several ways to find support groups for CKD patients. Your doctor, nephrologist, or healthcare team may have recommendations for local support groups in your area. Hospitals and kidney care centers often host regular group meetings where patients can come together to discuss their experiences and provide mutual support. These groups are typically led by healthcare professionals who can offer guidance on managing CKD.

Online support groups are another excellent option, especially if you're unable to attend in-person meetings. Online groups offer flexibility and accessibility, allowing you to connect with others from the comfort of your home. Many online forums and social media platforms, such as Facebook, offer CKD-specific support groups where patients and caregivers can share their stories, ask for advice, and offer emotional support.

Some reputable organizations that provide online support groups and forums for CKD patients include:

- **National Kidney Foundation (NKF):** Offers both in-person and online support through its NKF Peers Program, where people living with kidney disease can connect with trained peer mentors.
- **American Association of Kidney Patients (AAKP):** Provides access to educational materials, patient stories, and online support through the AAKP Patient Support Group.
- **Kidney Disease Improving Global Outcomes (KDIGO):** KDIGO offers resources, webinars, and support for patients and families dealing with CKD.

Engaging with these groups can help you feel more informed about your condition and provide a sense of community, knowing that others are facing similar challenges.

4. Talking to Loved Ones About Your Condition

Talking to family and friends about your CKD diagnosis can be challenging, especially when you're still processing it yourself. It's common to feel hesitant or unsure about how much to share, but honest communication is essential for building a supportive environment.

When discussing your diagnosis with loved ones, start by explaining what CKD is, how it affects you, and what your treatment plan looks like. Some people may not be familiar with the disease, so it's helpful to provide clear information. You can share details about any lifestyle changes you'll need to make, such as dietary restrictions, medications, or possible treatments like dialysis. Let them know how you're feeling, both physically and emotionally, so they can better understand the challenges you're facing.

As you share this information, it's important to express how they can support you. For example, if you're feeling anxious about upcoming medical appointments, ask if they can accompany you. If you're feeling isolated, invite them to spend time with you, whether it's going for a walk, watching a movie, or simply talking. Being specific about your needs helps them offer meaningful support.

Some loved ones may find it difficult to process the news or may not know how to respond. Give them time to adjust and encourage them to ask questions. The more open and communicative you are, the easier it will be for them to understand your condition and offer the support you need.

5. The Importance of Mental Health Counseling and Therapy

While support from family, friends, and peers is invaluable, sometimes professional help is needed to address the emotional impact of living with CKD. Mental health counseling or therapy can be highly beneficial for managing feelings of anxiety, depression, or stress that may arise from dealing with a chronic illness.

Talking to a therapist or counselor can help you explore your feelings in a safe, non-judgmental environment. They can provide tools and strategies to manage difficult emotions, cope with the challenges of CKD, and improve your overall mental health. Therapy can also be a space where you learn how to communicate more effectively with loved ones about your needs and emotions.

For some people, combining therapy with medication for anxiety or depression can be helpful. If you're struggling to manage your mental health, discuss this with your doctor. They can refer you to a mental health professional and help you explore treatment options that align with your needs. Therapies such as Cognitive Behavioral Therapy (CBT) are particularly effective for addressing the negative thought patterns that can lead to anxiety and depression. CBT helps you reframe negative thoughts into more positive, realistic ones, allowing you to better manage stress and emotional distress.

How to Talk to Loved Ones About Your Condition

Talking to your loved ones about your Chronic Kidney Disease (CKD) diagnosis can be one of the most challenging aspects of managing the disease, but it's an essential step in building a supportive network. Many people hesitate to share their diagnosis because they don't want to worry their family or friends, or they may not know how to communicate the seriousness of the condition without overwhelming others. However, open and honest conversations can bring you closer to your loved ones and help them understand how they can support you emotionally, physically, and practically.

In this section, we'll explore strategies for talking to your family and friends about CKD, how to explain the disease in a way that's understandable, and how to express your emotional and practical needs without feeling like a burden.

1. Preparing for the Conversation

Before you talk to your loved ones, take some time to reflect on what you want to communicate and how much you're comfortable sharing. The conversation doesn't have to happen all at once. You can share information in stages, starting with the basics of your diagnosis and gradually explaining the details of how CKD affects your life.

Think about how your diagnosis has impacted you both physically and emotionally, and consider what specific support you might need from those closest to you. Whether it's a listening ear, help with medical appointments, or assistance with daily tasks, being clear about your needs can make it easier for your loved ones to understand how to help.

You may also want to prepare for different reactions. Some people might be empathetic and ready to offer support, while others may need more time to process the information or might not know how to respond right away. It's important to be patient and understand that people may react in various ways, depending on their relationship with you and their own feelings about health issues.

2. Explaining Your Diagnosis in Simple Terms

When talking about CKD, it's helpful to explain the condition in straightforward, easy-to-understand terms. Start by explaining what CKD is and how it affects your kidneys. You might say, "Chronic Kidney Disease means that my kidneys aren't working as well as they should, and over time, this can get worse. I need to make some changes to my lifestyle and follow a treatment plan to keep things from getting worse."

You can then explain how CKD might affect your daily life. For example, you might mention that you need to be careful about what you eat, that you'll be taking certain medications, or that you'll need regular medical checkups to monitor your kidney function. If you have any symptoms like fatigue, swelling, or changes in urination, let your loved ones know how these symptoms impact your day-to-day routine.

If your loved ones have questions, answer them as openly as you feel comfortable, but remember that you don't have to share every detail if you're not ready. Focus on the key information they need to know, such as how the disease will affect you and what kind of support you might need from them.

3. Expressing Your Emotional Needs

Sharing the emotional impact of CKD with your loved ones is just as important as discussing the physical aspects of the disease. It's natural to feel a range of emotions after being diagnosed with CKD, including fear, sadness, frustration, and even anger. Your family and friends may not immediately understand how deeply the diagnosis has affected you unless you open up about your feelings.

You can begin by explaining how the diagnosis has made you feel. You might say, "This diagnosis has been really hard for me to process, and sometimes I feel overwhelmed or anxious about what's to come." Let your loved ones know that it helps to have someone listen when you're feeling down, and that talking about your feelings can be a relief.

If you're finding it difficult to talk about your emotions, it can be helpful to write down your thoughts beforehand or even share a letter or email with your loved ones. This gives you the opportunity to express yourself clearly without the pressure of face-to-face conversation, which can sometimes feel overwhelming.

4. Asking for Practical Help

In addition to emotional support, you may need practical help managing your CKD. Whether it's assistance with transportation to doctor's appointments, help with preparing kidney-friendly meals, or simply having someone to accompany you to medical consultations, asking for practical support can ease some of the stress that comes with managing a chronic illness.

When asking for help, it's important to be specific about what you need. Instead of saying, "I'm struggling to manage everything," try something more direct, like "I could really use some help with driving to my appointments, as it's hard for me to handle on my own." By being specific, your loved ones will know exactly how they can assist, and they're more likely to feel empowered to step in.

It's also helpful to let your loved ones know that their support makes a big difference. Many people want to help but may not know how. Expressing gratitude for their assistance can strengthen your bond and make them feel valued.

5. Balancing Your Independence with Support

While it's important to ask for help when you need it, you may also want to maintain a sense of independence as you manage your CKD. It's common to feel torn between wanting support and not wanting to burden your loved ones. However, finding a balance between independence and support is key to maintaining healthy relationships and managing your condition effectively.

Let your loved ones know that while you appreciate their help, you also value your independence. You might say, "I'm working on managing my CKD on my own as much as I can, but there are times when I'll need your support, and I'll let you know when that is." This allows you to retain autonomy while also giving your loved ones permission to step in when necessary.

6. Encouraging Open Communication

Your diagnosis is likely to raise concerns and questions among your loved ones, and they may not always know the best way to bring them up. Encouraging open communication ensures that everyone feels comfortable discussing the condition without fear of judgment or discomfort.

Let your family and friends know that they can come to you with any questions or concerns they have about your CKD. You can say, "If you ever have questions about my treatment or how I'm feeling, please don't hesitate to ask. I want to keep an open dialogue so we can all support each other."
This open approach fosters a sense of trust and transparency, allowing your loved ones to better understand what you're going through and how they can help.

7. Giving Loved Ones Time to Process
It's important to remember that your loved ones may need time to process your diagnosis. CKD can be a complex condition, and while you've had time to come to terms with it, they may be hearing the news for the first time. Some family members or friends may react with shock or concern, while others may take a more practical approach. Give them space to ask questions, express their feelings, and adjust to the news.
If you sense that someone is struggling to cope with your diagnosis, encourage them to seek support as well. It might be helpful for them to talk to a counselor or join a caregiver support group to process their own emotions about your condition.

The Importance of Mental Health Counseling and Therapy

Living with Chronic Kidney Disease (CKD) can take a toll not only on your physical health but also on your emotional well-being. The stress of managing a chronic illness, combined with the fear and uncertainty that often accompany such a diagnosis, can lead to feelings of anxiety, depression, and hopelessness. In addition to seeking support from loved ones and peer groups, professional mental health counseling and therapy can be invaluable in helping you cope with the emotional impact of CKD.

This section will explore the benefits of mental health counseling, how therapy can help manage anxiety and depression, and when you should consider seeking professional support.

1. Why Mental Health Counseling is Essential for CKD Patients

Chronic Kidney Disease is a life-altering condition that brings with it not only physical symptoms but also emotional and psychological challenges. The burden of dealing with a long-term illness, coupled with lifestyle changes, treatment plans, and the possibility of dialysis or a kidney transplant, can feel overwhelming. Many people with CKD experience stress, fear, anxiety, and depression at various stages of the disease. Mental health counseling provides a safe and confidential space to explore these feelings. A trained counselor or therapist can help you process your emotions, develop coping strategies, and work through any fears or concerns related to your diagnosis and treatment. Therapy also helps address the broader impact CKD can have on your life, such as changes in your relationships, work, or sense of independence.

In addition to providing emotional support, mental health counseling can help you improve your quality of life by addressing underlying issues that may interfere with your ability to manage CKD. For instance, depression can make it harder to follow through with dietary changes, medication schedules, or exercise routines. By treating the emotional aspects of CKD, counseling can improve your overall adherence to treatment and help you regain a sense of control.

2. Managing Anxiety and Depression Through Therapy

Anxiety and depression are two of the most common mental health issues that people with CKD face. The uncertainty of living with a chronic illness, the fear of disease progression, and the emotional toll of lifestyle adjustments can trigger feelings of intense worry, sadness, or hopelessness. These emotions can sometimes feel paralyzing, making it difficult to cope with daily life.

Therapy, especially Cognitive Behavioral Therapy (CBT), is an effective treatment for managing both anxiety and depression. CBT focuses on identifying and changing negative thought patterns that contribute to emotional distress. For example, if you find yourself constantly worrying about the future or feeling helpless about your CKD, a therapist can help you recognize these patterns and develop healthier ways of thinking.

In therapy, you'll learn practical tools to manage symptoms of anxiety and depression. These might include relaxation techniques, mindfulness practices, or behavioral strategies to improve your mood and reduce stress. Over time, therapy can help you feel more empowered in managing your CKD, making it easier to handle the emotional challenges that come with the disease.

For people dealing with severe anxiety or depression, therapy may also be combined with medication. Antidepressants or anti-anxiety medications can help stabilize your mood, making it easier to engage in therapy and follow through with treatment. Always consult with your healthcare provider before starting any medication to ensure it is safe and appropriate for your situation.

3. When to Seek Professional Help

While it's normal to feel sad or anxious at times, there are certain signs that indicate it might be time to seek professional mental health support. If you notice that feelings of anxiety or depression are interfering with your daily life or ability to manage your CKD, it's important to reach out for help.

Consider seeking counseling if you:
- Feel persistently sad, hopeless, or overwhelmed.
- . Have difficulty sleeping or find yourself sleeping too much.
- Experience a loss of interest in activities you once enjoyed.
- Find it hard to concentrate or make decisions.
- . Feel anxious or panicked about the future.

- Are struggling to keep up with your treatment plan or make healthy choices.
- Feel isolated or withdraw from family and friends.
- Experience thoughts of self-harm or suicide.

If you recognize any of these symptoms in yourself, therapy can provide a pathway to healing and help you regain a sense of balance. The sooner you seek support, the sooner you can begin working through these feelings and improve your mental health.

4. How to Find a Therapist

Finding the right therapist is an important step in managing the emotional impact of CKD. Many mental health professionals specialize in working with people who have chronic illnesses, and they can offer valuable insight into the specific challenges you're facing.

To find a therapist, you can start by asking your doctor for a referral. Many healthcare providers have relationships with mental health professionals who are experienced in working with patients managing chronic conditions like CKD. You can also check with your insurance company for a list of in-network therapists or use online directories like Psychology Today, which allows you to search for therapists based on location, specialty, and treatment approach.

If in-person therapy is not an option, many therapists now offer teletherapy, which allows you to meet with a therapist virtually. This can be especially helpful if you have mobility issues or live in a rural area where in-person services may not be available.

When choosing a therapist, it's important to find someone you feel comfortable with. You should feel safe and supported in therapy, and it's okay to try different therapists until you find the right fit. During your first few sessions, don't hesitate to ask questions about the therapist's experience, approach to treatment, and how they might help you manage the emotional aspects of CKD.

In some cases, CKD can strain relationships with family members or partners. The demands of managing a chronic illness can create stress within the family, leading to misunderstandings or conflict. Family counseling or couples therapy can be beneficial for navigating these challenges. In family counseling, a therapist works with you and your loved ones to improve communication and address any emotional issues related to the impact of CKD. Family members often have their own concerns and fears about your health, and counseling provides a space to express these feelings and work through them together. By fostering open communication, family counseling can strengthen your support system and improve your emotional well-being. For those in a romantic relationship, couples therapy can help address the unique challenges that CKD may bring to your partnership. Issues such as changes in physical health, emotional distance, or shifts in daily responsibilities can strain a relationship. Couples therapy can help both partners navigate these changes, ensuring that the relationship remains strong and supportive as you manage CKD together.

5. Integrating Mental Health Care into Your Overall Treatment Plan

Managing CKD involves a holistic approach that addresses both your physical and emotional health. Integrating mental health care into your overall treatment plan can significantly improve your ability to cope with the disease and enhance your quality of life.

During your medical appointments, don't hesitate to discuss your mental health with your doctor. They can help you determine whether counseling or therapy might be beneficial and can refer you to trusted mental health professionals. By addressing both the physical and emotional aspects of CKD, you'll have a stronger foundation for managing the disease and staying on track with your treatment plan.

It's also helpful to practice self-care as part of your mental health routine. This might include relaxation techniques like deep breathing or meditation, physical activities like walking or yoga, and hobbies that bring you joy and relaxation. Engaging in regular self-care can help reduce stress and anxiety, improving your overall well-being.

CHAPTER NINE

PREVENTING FURTHER KIDNEY DAMAGE

Preventing the Worsening of CKD

What You Can Do to Slow Down Disease Progression

Once you've been diagnosed with Chronic Kidney Disease (CKD), your focus should shift to managing the disease and taking steps to slow its progression. CKD progresses gradually, and in its early stages, you may not experience significant symptoms. However, taking proactive steps early can help protect your kidney function for as long as possible. Slowing the progression of CKD requires a combination of lifestyle changes, medication management, and regular monitoring by your healthcare team.

In this section, we'll explore the key strategies for slowing down CKD progression, including controlling underlying conditions, making dietary changes, and adopting healthy lifestyle habits.

1. Controlling Underlying Conditions

One of the most important steps in slowing CKD progression is managing any underlying health conditions that contribute to kidney damage. Two of the most common conditions that worsen CKD are diabetes and high blood pressure (hypertension). Both of these conditions can cause significant stress on the kidneys over time, and if left unmanaged, they can accelerate kidney damage.

If you have diabetes, maintaining good blood sugar control is critical. Elevated blood sugar levels can damage the blood vessels in the kidneys, leading to reduced kidney function. Work closely with your doctor to monitor your blood sugar levels and follow any dietary or medication recommendations designed to keep your glucose levels within a healthy range. Medications like insulin or oral diabetes medications may be necessary to help regulate your blood sugar.

For those with high blood pressure, it's essential to keep your blood pressure within a healthy range to reduce the strain on your kidneys. High blood pressure damages the small blood vessels in the kidneys, reducing their ability to filter waste from the blood. Medications such as ACE inhibitors or ARBs are often prescribed to help lower blood pressure and protect kidney function. Regular monitoring of your blood pressure, either at home or with your doctor, is important to ensure that your levels remain stable.

Other coexisting conditions, such as heart disease, can also worsen CKD. Managing your cardiovascular health through regular exercise, a heart-healthy diet, and medication (if needed) can help prevent further kidney damage. By keeping these conditions under control, you'll reduce the overall stress on your kidneys and slow disease progression.

2. Following a Kidney-Friendly Diet

Diet plays a critical role in managing CKD and protecting your remaining kidney function. Your kidneys are responsible for filtering waste products and excess fluid from your blood, and what you eat directly impacts how hard your kidneys must work. A kidney-friendly diet helps reduce the buildup of waste and toxins in the body, which in turn slows the progression of CKD.

One of the first dietary changes most people with CKD need to make is reducing sodium intake. High sodium levels can lead to fluid retention and increase blood pressure, both of which put extra strain on your kidneys. Aim to consume no more than 2,000 milligrams of sodium per day. This means avoiding processed foods, salty snacks, and restaurant meals, which are often high in hidden sodium. Instead, focus on whole foods like fresh vegetables, fruits, and lean proteins.

Controlling protein intake is another important aspect of a kidney-friendly diet. While your body needs protein to maintain muscle mass and support other functions, too much protein can produce waste products that your kidneys must filter. Depending on your stage of CKD, your doctor or dietitian may recommend limiting your protein intake to reduce the burden on your kidneys. High-quality protein sources, such as lean meats, fish, eggs, and plant-based proteins, are usually preferred over processed meats and high-fat proteins.

You may also need to limit potassium and phosphorus, particularly in the later stages of CKD. High potassium levels (hyperkalemia) can cause dangerous heart problems, while elevated phosphorus can lead to bone and heart complications. Foods high in potassium, such as bananas, potatoes, and tomatoes, may need to be limited, while phosphorus-rich foods like dairy products, nuts, and processed meats should also be restricted. Your doctor will help you determine your specific dietary needs based on your blood test results.

Finally, staying well-hydrated is important, but if your doctor has advised you to limit fluids due to advanced CKD, it's essential to follow their recommendations closely. Too much fluid can lead to swelling, high blood pressure, and additional strain on the kidneys.

3. Taking Medications as Prescribed

Medication management is a key component of slowing down CKD progression. Your doctor may prescribe medications to control blood pressure, manage blood sugar levels, reduce proteinuria (the presence of protein in your urine), and treat anemia or bone disease associated with CKD. It's crucial to take all medications as prescribed to keep your kidney function stable and prevent complications.

ACE inhibitors and ARBs are commonly prescribed to help reduce blood pressure and protect the kidneys. These medications work by relaxing blood vessels, reducing the workload on the kidneys, and lowering protein levels in the urine. Studies have shown that ACE inhibitors and ARBs can significantly slow the progression of CKD, particularly in people with diabetes or high blood pressure.

In some cases, your doctor may prescribe medications to manage high cholesterol or anemia. High cholesterol can lead to atherosclerosis (hardening of the arteries), which reduces blood flow to the kidneys and worsens CKD. Statins are often used to lower cholesterol levels and reduce cardiovascular risk. Erythropoiesis-stimulating agents (ESAs) may be used to treat anemia by stimulating the production of red blood cells, improving your energy levels and overall health.

It's also important to avoid certain over-the-counter medications that can damage your kidneys. Nonsteroidal anti-inflammatory drugs (NSAIDs), such as ibuprofen and naproxen, can worsen kidney function, especially when used long-term. Always consult your doctor before taking any new medications or supplements, and inform them of all medications you're currently taking to avoid potential drug interactions.

4. Regular Monitoring and Early Intervention

One of the most effective ways to slow CKD progression is through regular monitoring of your kidney function and addressing any changes early. Your doctor will use blood and urine tests to track how well your kidneys are filtering waste and managing fluid levels. Key tests include serum creatinine, glomerular filtration rate (GFR), and urine albuminlevels. These tests help your healthcare provider determine whether your CKD is stable or worsening and guide treatment adjustments as needed.

Early intervention is critical in preventing further kidney damage. If your doctor detects a decline in kidney function, they may adjust your medications, recommend dietary changes, or suggest other treatments to slow the progression of the disease. Catching changes early can prevent more serious complications down the road, such as the need for dialysis or a kidney transplant.

It's important to attend all scheduled medical appointments and follow up with your doctor regularly, even if you're feeling well. CKD can progress silently, and monitoring your kidney function through regular tests ensures that any changes are detected and treated early.

5. Adopting a Healthy Lifestyle

In addition to managing your diet and medications, adopting a healthy lifestyle is essential for slowing CKD progression and protecting your overall health. Physical activity is beneficial for maintaining a healthy weight, improving cardiovascular health, and reducing blood pressure. Aim for at least 30 minutes of moderate exercise, such as walking, swimming, or cycling, most days of the week. Exercise not only helps protect your kidneys but also improves your energy levels and mental well-being.

Quitting smoking is one of the most important lifestyle changes you can make to protect your kidneys. Smoking damages blood vessels and reduces blood flow to the kidneys, accelerating kidney damage. If you smoke, talk to your doctor about smoking cessation programs or medications that can help you quit.

Managing stress is also important for kidney health. Chronic stress can raise blood pressure and increase the risk of heart disease, both of which can worsen CKD. Practice stress-relief techniques like deep breathing exercises, meditation, or yoga to help keep your stress levels in check.

Managing Coexisting Conditions Like Diabetes and Hypertension

Managing Chronic Kidney Disease (CKD) often involves addressing coexisting conditions that can exacerbate kidney damage. Two of the most common conditions associated with CKD are diabetes and hypertension (high blood pressure), both of which can significantly impact the progression of kidney disease. Successfully controlling these conditions is critical for protecting your kidneys and slowing the advancement of CKD.

In this section, we will explain how diabetes and hypertension affect kidney health, and the steps you can take to manage these conditions and protect your kidney function.

1. Diabetes and CKD

Diabetes is one of the leading causes of CKD. High blood sugar levels over time can damage the small blood vessels in the kidneys, impairing their ability to filter waste from the blood. This condition, known as diabetic nephropathy, can worsen CKD and lead to further complications like high blood pressure and heart disease.

For individuals with diabetes, managing blood sugar levels is crucial in slowing the progression of CKD. Good blood sugar control can help reduce the damage to the kidneys and improve overall kidney health. Here are some key strategies for managing diabetes and protecting your kidneys:

Monitor blood sugar levels regularly: Keeping a close eye on your blood sugar levels allows you to detect any spikes or dips early. Your healthcare provider may recommend daily glucose monitoring to ensure your levels stay within a healthy range.

Follow a diabetes-friendly diet: A balanced diet is essential for managing blood sugar. Focus on whole grains, lean proteins, and non-starchy vegetables while limiting refined carbohydrates, sugary foods, and saturated fats. Your doctor or dietitian can help design a meal plan tailored to your needs.

Take medications as prescribed: Many people with diabetes require medications such as insulin or oral diabetes medications to help control blood sugar levels. It's important to take these medications as directed to avoid complications that can further damage your kidneys.

Exercise regularly: Physical activity helps lower blood sugar levels and improve insulin sensitivity. Aim for at least 30 minutes of moderate exercise, such as walking or swimming, on most days of the week. This can improve blood sugar control and reduce the strain on your kidneys.

Manage stress: Stress can cause blood sugar levels to fluctuate, making it harder to control diabetes. Incorporate relaxation techniques like meditation, yoga, or deep breathing into your daily routine to manage stress.

By taking steps to manage diabetes effectively, you can reduce the impact it has on your kidneys and slow the progression of CKD.

2. Hypertension and CKD

Hypertension (high blood pressure) is another major contributor to CKD progression. High blood pressure damages the blood vessels in the kidneys, reducing their ability to filter waste effectively. Over time, untreated hypertension can lead to further kidney damage, accelerating the progression to end-stage renal disease (ESRD) and increasing the risk of heart disease.

Managing blood pressure is one of the most important ways to protect your kidneys. Here are some strategies for controlling hypertension and supporting kidney health:

Monitor your blood pressure regularly: If you have high blood pressure, regular monitoring is essential. Your doctor may recommend using a home blood pressure monitor to track your levels between appointments. Keeping your blood pressure within the target range (usually around 120/80 mmHg) is key to preventing further kidney damage.

Follow a low-sodium diet: Reducing sodium intake helps lower blood pressure and reduce fluid retention, which can ease the strain on your kidneys. Aim for less than 2,000 milligrams of sodium per day by avoiding processed foods, canned goods, and salty snacks. Use herbs and spices to flavor your meals instead of salt.

Take blood pressure medications as prescribed: Many people with CKD and hypertension need medications to help control their blood pressure. Common medications include ACE inhibitors or ARBs, which not only lower blood pressure but also protect the kidneys by reducing protein levels in the urine. It's important to take these medications as directed and work with your doctor to adjust doses as needed.

Stay physically active: Regular exercise helps lower blood pressure and improves cardiovascular health. Aim for moderate-intensity activities like walking, cycling, or swimming for at least 150 minutes per week. Physical activity can also help you manage stress, another factor that contributes to high blood pressure.

Maintain a healthy weight: Excess weight puts additional strain on your heart and kidneys. Losing even a small amount of weight can help lower blood pressure and improve kidney function. Talk to your doctor or a dietitian about developing a weight management plan that's safe and effective for you.

3. The Link Between Diabetes, Hypertension, and CKD

Diabetes and hypertension are closely linked, and many people with CKD have both conditions. High blood sugar levels and elevated blood pressure can work together to damage the kidneys more quickly. This is why it's especially important for individuals with both diabetes and hypertension to manage these conditions aggressively.

By controlling blood sugar and blood pressure simultaneously, you can reduce the overall burden on your kidneys and slow the progression of CKD. Regular check-ups with your healthcare provider, combined with lifestyle changes and medications, can help keep both conditions under control and prevent further kidney damage.

4. Regular Monitoring and Early Intervention

For people managing CKD alongside diabetes and hypertension, regular monitoring of blood pressure, blood sugar levels, and kidney function is essential. Your healthcare team will monitor key markers like creatinine, GFR, and albumin levels to assess your kidney function and determine whether any adjustments to your treatment plan are necessary.

Early intervention is critical to preventing further kidney damage. If your healthcare provider notices a decline in kidney function or an increase in blood pressure or blood sugar levels, they can adjust your medications or recommend lifestyle changes to get these conditions under control. Addressing issues early can prevent them from worsening and help protect your remaining kidney function.

5. The Role of Medication in Managing Coexisting Conditions

Medications play a crucial role in managing diabetes, hypertension, and CKD. In addition to medications that directly target kidney function, you may need drugs to control blood sugar, blood pressure, and cholesterol. Managing all of these factors helps reduce the strain on your kidneys and prevent complications like heart disease.

Your doctor may prescribe medications such as:

a. ACE inhibitors or ARBs to lower blood pressure and protect kidney function.

b. Diuretics to help remove excess fluid and reduce blood pressure.

c. Insulin or oral diabetes medications to control blood sugar levels.

d. Statins to manage high cholesterol, which can worsen kidney disease and increase the risk of heart problems.

It's important to take all prescribed medications as directed and discuss any side effects with your doctor. Regular follow-ups will help ensure that your medications are working effectively and that adjustments are made as needed.

The Role of Early Intervention

Why Starting Treatment Early Can Help Save Your Kidneys
Early treatment is crucial when it comes to managing Chronic Kidney Disease (CKD). The earlier CKD is detected and treated, the better your chances of slowing its progression and protecting your remaining kidney function. CKD often progresses gradually and, in its early stages, can be asymptomatic. This is why many people are unaware they have CKD until significant kidney damage has already occurred. Starting treatment early, even before symptoms appear, can make a significant difference in long-term outcomes.

CKD progresses in stages, and without intervention, it can lead to more severe complications, including end-stage kidney disease (ESKD), where dialysis or a kidney transplant becomes necessary. By initiating treatment as soon as CKD is diagnosed, you can prevent further kidney damage and extend the functionality of your kidneys for as long as possible.

1. Detecting CKD Early

One of the biggest challenges in managing CKD is that it often goes undetected in the early stages. Routine blood and urine tests are the best tools for detecting CKD before significant symptoms develop. Tests such as creatinine levels, glomerular filtration rate (GFR), and urine albumin-to-creatinine ratio can reveal how well your kidneys are functioning and whether there are early signs of damage.

If you are at risk for CKD due to factors like high blood pressure, diabetes, or a family history of kidney disease, it's essential to undergo regular testing. Early detection allows your healthcare provider to develop a treatment plan that addresses the underlying causes of CKD and prevents further damage.

2. Reducing Risk Factors Early On

When CKD is detected early, the focus of treatment is on reducing the factors that contribute to kidney damage. For instance, controlling high blood pressure and blood sugar levels can dramatically slow the progression of CKD. Uncontrolled hypertension and diabetes are two of the leading causes of kidney damage, and addressing these conditions promptly helps reduce the strain on your kidneys.

By starting treatment early, you can also make critical lifestyle changes, such as following a kidney-friendly diet, limiting salt and protein intake, and staying active. These steps are easier to implement when CKD is still in its early stages, giving your kidneys the best chance to remain functional for as long as possible.

3. Preventing Complications

CKD can lead to a variety of complications, including anemia, bone disease, and cardiovascular problems. These complications become more difficult to manage as the disease progresses, which is why early treatment is key. By starting treatment early, your healthcare provider can monitor and address these potential complications before they become severe.

For example, CKD-related anemia occurs when the kidneys can no longer produce enough of the hormone erythropoietin, which stimulates red blood cell production. By detecting this condition early, doctors can prescribe treatments like erythropoiesis-stimulating agents (ESAs) or iron supplements to manage anemia and improve your overall quality of life.

Similarly, early treatment can help prevent bone disease, which occurs when the kidneys fail to properly regulate calcium and phosphorus levels in the body. By addressing these imbalances early, doctors can prevent bone weakening and reduce the risk of fractures.

4. Preserving Kidney Function

One of the primary goals of early CKD treatment is to preserve as much kidney function as possible. Even in the early stages of CKD, small changes to your treatment plan can significantly reduce the workload on your kidneys and protect their function over time. Medications, dietary adjustments, and lifestyle changes all contribute to preserving your kidney function.

Early use of medications like ACE inhibitors or ARBs can reduce blood pressure and protein levels in the urine, both of which are critical for protecting your kidneys. These medications are often prescribed in the early stages of CKD, as studies have shown they can significantly slow the progression of kidney disease and reduce the risk of reaching end-stage renal disease (ESRD).

5. Delaying the Need for Dialysis or Transplant

One of the most significant benefits of starting CKD treatment early is the ability to delay, or even prevent, the need for dialysis or a kidney transplant. Dialysis and transplants are necessary when kidney function falls below a critical level, but with early intervention, it's possible to extend kidney function and delay these treatments for many years.

By taking proactive steps to manage your condition, you can often avoid the complications that lead to rapid kidney deterioration. The earlier you start treatment, the more time you give yourself to manage the disease effectively and maintain a better quality of life.

How to Recognize Early Warning Signs of Kidney Deterioration

Recognizing the early warning signs of kidney deterioration is essential in managing Chronic Kidney Disease (CKD) and preventing further damage. While CKD often progresses silently in its early stages, there are specific symptoms and changes that can indicate worsening kidney function. By being vigilant about these signs and staying proactive with regular medical checkups, you can catch problems early and take action before the disease progresses to a more advanced stage.

In this section, we'll be discussing the key symptoms to watch for, how to monitor your health, and the importance of regular testing in detecting early signs of kidney deterioration.

1. Fatigue and Weakness

One of the most common early signs of worsening kidney function is persistent fatigue and weakness. As your kidneys lose their ability to filter waste and excess fluids from your blood, toxins can build up, leading to feelings of tiredness and a general lack of energy. This can make it harder to complete daily tasks or stay active, and you might find that you feel more exhausted than usual, even after getting plenty of rest.

Fatigue can also be a sign of anemia, a condition that often develops in the later stages of CKD. When the kidneys aren't functioning properly, they produce less of the hormone erythropoietin, which stimulates red blood cell production. Without enough red blood cells to carry oxygen to your tissues, you may feel tired and weak. If you're experiencing unexplained fatigue, it's important to talk to your doctor, as early intervention can help manage anemia and improve your energy levels.

2. Changes in Urination

Your kidneys play a central role in producing urine and removing waste from the body, so changes in urination are often one of the first signs that something is wrong. Pay attention to any changes in the frequency, color, or amount of urine you produce, as these can indicate kidney deterioration.

Some key changes to watch for include:

Increased or decreased urination: If you notice that you're urinating much more or much less than usual, it could be a sign that your kidneys are struggling to balance fluids and waste in your body.

Foamy or bubbly urine: This can be a sign of protein in the urine (proteinuria), which indicates that your kidneys are leaking protein and not filtering waste properly.

Dark-colored urine: Urine that is darker than normal or has a reddish-brown tint can indicate the presence of blood, which is a sign of kidney damage.

Frequent nighttime urination (nocturia): Waking up multiple times during the night to urinate can be a sign of worsening kidney function, as your kidneys may be struggling to balance fluids during the day.

If you notice any of these changes in your urination patterns, it's important to consult your doctor as soon as possible. They can perform tests to determine whether your kidneys are functioning properly and recommend appropriate treatment.

3. Swelling (Edema)

Another early warning sign of kidney deterioration is swelling or edema, which occurs when your kidneys are unable to remove excess fluid from your body. This fluid buildup can cause noticeable swelling in your legs, ankles, feet, hands, or face. Swelling can be mild at first but may worsen over time as kidney function declines.

If you notice persistent or unexplained swelling, particularly in your lower extremities, it's important to bring this up with your healthcare provider. Edema can also be caused by other conditions, such as heart disease or liver problems, so it's important to get a proper diagnosis to determine the underlying cause.

4. Shortness of Breath

As CKD progresses and your kidneys become less effective at removing waste and fluid, shortness of breath can develop. This occurs when excess fluid builds up in the lungs, making it harder to breathe. You may notice that you feel short of breath after physical activity or even while resting.

Shortness of breath can also be related to anemia, as your body may not be getting enough oxygen due to a reduced red blood cell count. If you're experiencing breathing difficulties, it's essential to seek medical attention right away, as this could be a sign of worsening kidney function or other complications that need immediate treatment.

5. High Blood Pressure

High blood pressure is both a cause and a symptom of CKD. As your kidneys become damaged, they have a harder time regulating blood pressure, which can lead to hypertension. Conversely, uncontrolled high blood pressure can also damage the blood vessels in your kidneys, accelerating kidney deterioration.

If you've already been diagnosed with high blood pressure, it's important to monitor your levels regularly and follow your doctor's recommendations for managing it. If you notice that your blood pressure is consistently higher than normal, despite taking medications or making lifestyle changes, it could be a sign that your kidneys are struggling to function properly. In this case, your doctor may need to adjust your treatment plan to better manage your blood pressure and protect your kidneys.

6. Nausea and Loss of Appetite

As kidney function declines, waste products can accumulate in your blood, leading to a condition known as uremia. Uremia can cause a variety of symptoms, including nausea, vomiting, and loss of appetite. You may notice that you feel less hungry than usual or that certain foods no longer appeal to you. Some people with CKD also experience a metallic taste in their mouth, which can further decrease their appetite.

If you're losing weight unintentionally or struggling to maintain a healthy diet due to nausea or lack of appetite, it's important to speak with your healthcare provider. They can help you manage these symptoms and ensure that you're getting the nutrients you need to support your overall health and kidney function.

7. Regular Monitoring and Early Intervention

While recognizing the early warning signs of kidney deterioration is important, regular medical monitoring is essential for detecting changes in kidney function before symptoms appear. Your healthcare provider will likely recommend regular blood and urine tests to track your kidney health and catch any signs of deterioration early.

Tests such as creatinine, glomerular filtration rate (GFR), and albumin-to-creatinine ratio can provide valuable insights into how well your kidneys are functioning. By detecting changes in these markers early, your doctor can adjust your treatment plan and take steps to slow the progression of CKD.

Early intervention is critical to preventing further kidney damage and managing complications. If you notice any changes in your symptoms or overall health, don't hesitate to reach out to your healthcare provider for advice and guidance.

Protecting Your Remaining Kidney Function

Lifestyle Habits to Maintain Kidney Health Over Time

When living with Chronic Kidney Disease (CKD), adopting and maintaining healthy lifestyle habits can significantly slow the progression of the disease and improve your overall quality of life. While medical treatment and regular monitoring are essential, making changes to your daily routine can help preserve kidney function and prevent complications. In this section, we will discuss the key lifestyle habits that support kidney health over time, including nutrition, exercise, hydration, and stress management.

1. Following a Kidney-Friendly Diet

One of the most critical aspects of managing CKD is maintaining a kidney-friendly diet. What you eat directly affects how hard your kidneys must work to filter waste and balance electrolytes in your body. A diet tailored to CKD helps reduce the buildup of waste products and fluid retention, making it easier for your kidneys to function effectively.

Here are some key dietary principles to follow for maintaining kidney health:

Limit sodium intake: Excess sodium can lead to high blood pressure, fluid retention, and swelling, which all put additional strain on your kidneys. Aim to consume less than 2,000 milligrams of sodium per day. Choose fresh, whole foods over processed options, and use herbs and spices to flavor your meals instead of salt.

Manage protein intake: While protein is essential for maintaining muscle mass, too much can increase the workload on your kidneys. Depending on your stage of CKD, your doctor or dietitian may recommend reducing your protein intake to prevent further kidney damage. Focus on high-quality proteins like lean meats, eggs, and plant-based proteins, and avoid excessive consumption of processed meats.

Control potassium and phosphorus levels: As CKD progresses, your kidneys may have difficulty regulating potassium and phosphorus levels. High potassium can lead to heart problems, while elevated phosphorus can weaken your bones. Your healthcare provider will guide you on which foods to limit based on your specific blood test results. Common potassium-rich foods to watch include bananas, tomatoes, and potatoes, while phosphorus can be found in dairy products, nuts, and processed foods.

Stay hydrated but manage fluid intake: Drinking water is important for kidney health, but if your doctor has advised you to limit fluids due to advanced CKD, it's essential to follow those recommendations carefully. Overhydration can lead to swelling and high blood pressure. Ask your doctor how much fluid you should consume each day and plan your intake accordingly.

2. Staying Physically Active

Regular physical activity is crucial for maintaining kidney health and supporting overall well-being. Exercise helps control blood pressure, reduce stress, manage weight, and improve cardiovascular health, all of which are important factors in slowing the progression of CKD.

Aim for at least 30 minutes of moderate exercise most days of the week. Activities such as walking, cycling, swimming, and yoga are excellent options, as they provide cardiovascular benefits without putting excessive strain on your body. If you're new to exercise or have mobility limitations, start with short, gentle activities and gradually increase the intensity and duration over time.

In addition to aerobic exercises, strength training can help maintain muscle mass, which can be affected by CKD. Simple bodyweight exercises, resistance band workouts, or light weightlifting can help you build strength without overexerting yourself.

Always check with your healthcare provider before starting a new exercise routine to ensure it's safe and suitable for your condition.

2. Managing Stress

Chronic stress can negatively impact kidney health by raising blood pressure, increasing inflammation, and contributing to overall feelings of anxiety or depression. Managing stress effectively is essential for preserving both mental and physical health while living with CKD.

Incorporating stress-reduction techniques into your daily routine can help you stay calm and focused, even when managing a chronic illness. Some helpful strategies include:

Mindfulness meditation: Practicing mindfulness helps you stay grounded in the present moment and reduce anxiety about the future. Set aside a few minutes each day to focus on your breathing and let go of any worries or stress.

Deep breathing exercises: Deep, controlled breathing can activate your body's relaxation response and lower blood pressure. When feeling stressed, take a few minutes to practice deep breathing by inhaling slowly through your nose, holding your breath for a few seconds, and exhaling slowly through your mouth.

Physical activity: Exercise is a proven way to reduce stress and boost your mood. Regular physical activity releases endorphins, which help alleviate stress and improve mental clarity.

Hobbies and relaxation: Make time for activities that bring you joy, whether it's reading, gardening, painting, or spending time with loved ones. Engaging in hobbies can provide a mental break from the demands of managing CKD.

4. Quitting Smoking and Limiting Alcohol

Smoking is a major risk factor for both kidney disease and cardiovascular disease, as it reduces blood flow to the kidneys and damages blood vessels. If you smoke, quitting is one of the most impactful steps you can take to protect your kidneys and improve your overall health. Smoking cessation programs, nicotine replacement therapies, and medications are available to help you quit, and your healthcare provider can guide you through the process.

Limiting alcohol is also important for people with CKD. Excessive alcohol consumption can raise blood pressure, worsen dehydration, and contribute to liver damage, all of which can strain the kidneys. If you choose to drink, do so in moderation, and discuss with your doctor how much is safe for your specific condition.

5. Maintaining a Healthy Weight

Being overweight or obese can worsen CKD by increasing the strain on your kidneys and raising your risk for other health problems, such as high blood pressure and diabetes. Maintaining a healthy weight through a balanced diet and regular exercise can reduce the workload on your kidneys and improve your overall health.

If you need to lose weight, aim for gradual, sustainable weight loss by making small changes to your diet and activity levels. Focus on eating nutrient-rich, whole foods and increasing your daily movement, whether through structured exercise or simple activities like walking more or taking the stairs.

6. Regular Medical Checkups and Monitoring

One of the most important lifestyle habits for managing CKD is staying consistent with your medical appointments and regular monitoring. Your healthcare provider will track your kidney function through blood and urine tests, monitor your blood pressure, and assess your overall health. These appointments allow your doctor to catch any changes in kidney function early and adjust your treatment plan as needed.

CHAPTER TEN

STORIES OF SUCCESS: PEOPLE WHO HAVE MANAGED CKD FOR YEARS.

Living with Chronic Kidney Disease (CKD) can feel overwhelming, but many individuals have successfully managed the condition for years, leading full and active lives. Their stories of perseverance and determination offer hope and inspiration to others navigating the challenges of CKD. Through a combination of medical treatment, lifestyle changes, and support from loved ones, these individuals have been able to slow the progression of the disease, maintain their quality of life, and, in some cases, even avoid dialysis or a kidney transplant for longer than expected.

In this section, we will share a few stories of success from people who have managed CKD over the long term. These personal accounts illustrate the power of proactive healthcare, positive attitudes, and persistence in overcoming the challenges that come with CKD.

1. Jane and thriving with CKD Through Early Intervention

Jane was diagnosed with stage 3 CKD at the age of 52 after a routine blood test revealed elevated creatinine levels. Although she was initially shocked and frightened by the diagnosis, Jane decided to take control of her health and work closely with her healthcare team to manage her condition.

Early intervention played a significant role in Jane's success. By making changes to her diet, including reducing sodium and protein intake, she was able to ease the strain on her kidneys. She also began taking medications to control her blood pressure and prevent further kidney damage. Regular exercise became an integral part of her routine, helping her maintain a healthy weight and improve her cardiovascular health.

With consistent medical monitoring and a commitment to following her treatment plan, Jane has successfully managed CKD for over 15 years. She continues to work with her doctors to adjust her treatment as needed and remains active, walking several miles a day and engaging in hobbies that keep her mind and body healthy.

2. David's story on managing CKD Alongside Diabetes

David was diagnosed with type 2 diabetes in his early 40s, and about ten years later, he learned that he also had CKD. At the time of his CKD diagnosis, David's kidney function was at stage 3, and his doctors informed him that his diabetes had likely contributed to the development of CKD.

Instead of becoming discouraged, David made the decision to take control of both his diabetes and CKD. By working closely with his doctor and dietitian, he learned how to balance his blood sugar levels and follow a kidney-friendly diet. He switched to high-quality protein sources, reduced his sodium intake, and cut out sugary foods that worsened his diabetes.

David also became diligent about taking his medications, including those prescribed to control his blood sugar and protect his kidneys. By keeping his blood pressure and blood sugar within target ranges, David has been able to significantly slow the progression of CKD. More than a decade after his diagnosis, his kidney function remains stable, and he has avoided the need for dialysis or a kidney transplant.

David attributes his success to early intervention, discipline, and regular checkups. He encourages others living with CKD to stay proactive in managing their health and not to be discouraged by the challenges of living with a chronic illness.

3. Maria's Success

Maria was diagnosed with end-stage kidney disease in her early 50s, after managing CKD for several years. When her kidney function declined to the point that dialysis was necessary, Maria underwent peritoneal dialysis at home for several months while she waited for a kidney transplant.

After receiving a kidney transplant, Maria's life changed dramatically. She was determined to make the most of her new kidney and live life to the fullest. By following her doctors' recommendations for immunosuppressive therapy, maintaining a strict medication regimen, and adopting a healthy lifestyle, Maria has successfully managed her condition post-transplant for over 10 years.

Maria continues to monitor her kidney function through regular follow-up appointments and stays vigilant about potential signs of organ rejection. She's grateful for the gift of her new kidney and works hard to protect it through good health habits, including eating a balanced diet, staying active, and avoiding anything that could harm her transplanted kidney.

Maria's story highlights the possibility of living a long and healthy life after a kidney transplant, provided that patients take care of their new organs and stay proactive about their health.

4. Peter's Story

Peter was diagnosed with stage 4 CKD in his mid-60s, after years of managing high blood pressure. As a busy professional and family man, Peter initially struggled to find balance between his demanding career, family life, and the need to manage his CKD.

With the help of his healthcare team, Peter developed a treatment plan that included regular medical checkups, blood pressure medications, and lifestyle changes to protect his kidneys. He learned how to manage his work stress through meditation and deep breathing exercises, which also helped lower his blood pressure. He prioritized spending time with his family, finding ways to stay connected to his loved ones without overextending himself.

Peter also made time for exercise, incorporating walks into his daily routine, and adjusted his diet to include kidney-friendly foods. Over time, he found a balance that allowed him to continue working and being present for his family while managing his CKD.

Now in his 70s, Peter's kidney function has remained stable, and he has avoided dialysis through a combination of medication, lifestyle changes, and stress management. His story is a testament to the power of finding balance and making small, sustainable changes that can have a lasting impact on health.

5. Sarah's Journey

Sarah was diagnosed with CKD in her late 40s, and like many people, she felt overwhelmed and isolated at first. However, through the support of an online CKD community, Sarah found strength and guidance from others who were living with the same condition. She joined a local support group where she could talk openly about her fears, challenges, and triumphs.

Through the guidance of her healthcare provider and the encouragement of her CKD community, Sarah learned how to manage her condition more effectively. She began following a kidney-friendly diet, exercising regularly, and keeping up with her medical appointments. The sense of connection and shared experience from her support group gave her the confidence to advocate for herself and make informed decisions about her health.

Sarah has managed CKD for over 12 years and continues to participate in online forums and local group meetings. She credits the support of her CKD community for helping her stay positive and motivated, even on the tough days. Sarah's journey highlights the importance of connecting with others who understand your experience and finding strength in community.

CONCLUSION

Reclaiming Your Health with CKD

Being diagnosed with Chronic Kidney Disease (CKD) can feel overwhelming, but it doesn't mean you've lost control over your health or future. With the right mindset, proactive care, and support, you can manage CKD and continue living a fulfilling, healthy life. This journey involves understanding your condition, making lifestyle changes, and working closely with your healthcare team to protect your kidneys and overall well-being.

By reclaiming your health with CKD, you are taking the reins of your treatment plan, making informed choices, and empowering yourself to stay active and engaged in life. You've learned that early intervention, consistent monitoring, and healthy habits can make a significant difference in slowing disease progression and improving quality of life.

How to Take Control of Your Kidney Health and Live Fully

Taking control of your kidney health begins with educating yourself about the disease and understanding the impact it has on your body. Knowing what to expect and how to manage CKD gives you the tools to make the best decisions for your health. Regular medical checkups, adherence to your treatment plan, and open communication with your healthcare provider are key steps to staying on top of your kidney function.

By adopting kidney-friendly lifestyle habits—such as following a balanced diet, exercising regularly, managing stress, and quitting smoking—you can preserve your kidney function and prevent complications. These changes may seem challenging at first, but they are essential for protecting your health and living life to the fullest.

Support is a crucial part of this journey. Whether you find encouragement from family, friends, or CKD support groups, having a strong network around you can make managing CKD easier. Don't be afraid to lean on others, share your concerns, or seek professional help when needed. Your emotional well-being is just as important as your physical health.

Moving Forward with Confidence and Hope

Managing CKD is a lifelong commitment, but it's a journey that you don't have to face alone. By focusing on what you can control—such as your lifestyle choices, medications, and regular monitoring—you can slow the progression of CKD and maintain a high quality of life. Advances in medical treatments and research are offering new hope for people with CKD, and staying informed about these developments will empower you to make the best choices for your future.

Approach each day with confidence and the understanding that you have the tools and resources to manage CKD. While the road may have challenges, it's filled with opportunities for growth, resilience, and hope. With a positive mindset and a proactive approach to your health, you can move forward with the knowledge that CKD does not define you or limit your potential for a healthy, fulfilling life.

Appendices

Glossary of Kidney Disease Terms

To help you better understand the medical language associated with CKD, here is a glossary of common terms:

- Albumin: A protein found in the blood. The presence of albumin in the urine can be a sign of kidney damage.

- Creatinine: A waste product produced by muscles that is filtered by the kidneys. High creatinine levels in the blood indicate reduced kidney function.

- Dialysis: A treatment that removes waste products and excess fluid from the blood when the kidneys can no longer perform this function.

- Glomerular Filtration Rate (GFR): A test that measures how well the kidneys are filtering waste from the blood. It is used to determine the stage of CKD.

- Hypertension: High blood pressure, which is both a cause and a result of kidney disease.

- Nephrologist: A doctor who specializes in diagnosing and treating kidney diseases.

- Proteinuria: The presence of excess protein in the urine, often a sign of kidney damage.

- Uremia: A condition that occurs when waste products build up in the blood due to kidney failure, leading to symptoms such as fatigue, nausea, and confusion.

Resources for CKD Patients

Knowledge and support are vital for managing CKD effectively. Below are some recommended resources that provide information, guidance, and community support for CKD patients:

Websites:

- National Kidney Foundation (NKF): www.kidney.org

- American Association of Kidney Patients (AAKP): www.aakp.org

- Renal Support Network (RSN): www.rsnhope.org

- Kidney Disease: Improving Global Outcomes (KDIGO): www.kdigo.org

Books:

- The Kidney Disease Solution by Duncan Capicchiano: A comprehensive guide to managing kidney disease naturally.

- Living Well with Kidney Failure by Juliet Auer: Offers advice for managing dialysis, kidney transplants, and CKD.

- Coping with Kidney Disease: A 12-Step Treatment Program to Help You Avoid Dialysis by Mackenzie Walser: Provides strategies for managing CKD in its early stages.

Organizations:

- National Kidney Foundation (NKF): Provides educational resources, patient support, and advocacy for kidney health.

- American Kidney Fund (AKF): Offers financial assistance to patients with kidney disease and provides resources for treatment and prevention.

- American Association of Kidney Patients (AAKP): A patient-led organization offering support, education, and advocacy for kidney disease patients.

Tracking Your Kidney Health

Staying organized and keeping track of your symptoms, medications, and test results can help you stay on top of your CKD management. Regular monitoring allows you to notice any changes in your health and communicate effectively with your healthcare provider.

- **Symptom Journal:** Keep a journal of any new or worsening symptoms you experience, such as changes in urination, fatigue, swelling, or shortness of breath. Noting the frequency and intensity of these symptoms can help your doctor adjust your treatment plan.

- **Medication Log:** Use a medication log to track when you take your medications, including dosage and any side effects. This helps ensure that you follow your treatment plan consistently and can address any concerns with your doctor.

- **Lab Results Tracker:** Record your blood and urine test results, such as GFR, creatinine, and albumin levels, over time. This will help you see trends in your kidney function and give you a clearer understanding of how your CKD is progressing.

By actively tracking your health and treatment, you can stay more informed and empowered in managing CKD. Regularly updating these records will help you stay organized and give you and your healthcare team valuable insights into your condition.

www.ingramcontent.com/pod-product-compliance
Lightning Source LLC
Chambersburg PA
CBHW071625220526
45469CB00002B/479